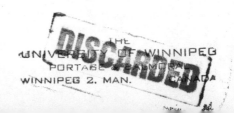

Allied Health Manpower:
Trends and Prospects

Allied Health Manpower:
Trends and Prospects

HARRY I. GREENFIELD

With the assistance of
CAROL A. BROWN

Foreword by
ELI GINZBERG

COLUMBIA UNIVERSITY PRESS
NEW YORK AND LONDON 1969

This report was prepared for the Manpower Administration, U.S. Department of Labor, under research contract Numbers 26231–26244 authorized by Title I of the Manpower Development and Training Act. Since contractors performing research under government sponsorship are encouraged to express their own judgment freely, the report does not necessarily represent the department's official opinion or policy. Moreover, the contractor is solely responsible for the factual accuracy of all material developed in the report.

Foreword

THE DRAMA OF MEDICINE is centered around the physician who, from the depth of his expertise, can diagnose the cause of the patient's illness and act to relieve his symptoms by removing the causes of his disability. This is how the layman sees the situation and this is how the physician has helped him to understand contemporary medicine.

But the facts are somewhat different. One of the important contributions that Harry Greenfield and Carol Brown have made in their new book, *Allied Health Manpower: Trends and Prospects,* is to provide a comprehensive view of the manpower dimensions of contemporary American medicine and, without denigrating the strategic role of the physician, to shed new light on the approximately 2.5 million persons who, together with the slightly more than 300,000 physicians, are engaged in the provision of health services. The authors are not primarily concerned with the relatively small numbers of independent practitioners such as dentists and other core professionals, nor even with the approximately 300,000 allied health professionals who have been trained between the baccalaureate and the doctoral levels and who fill such critical positions as bacteriologist, mycologist, biostatistician, virologist, hospital administrator, or clinical psychologist. Rather, their focus is on the approximately 1.7 million health workers who have been categorized as "allied health manpower," a reflection of the fact that they have one characteristic in common: all of them have had less than a full college education. While the majority are high-school graduates with some college training, a sizable number, probably over half a million, have not finished high school.

The single largest sub-group within allied health manpower are registered nurses who have graduated from a diploma school or from a junior college. They account for over half a million. But since nursing has been repeatedly singled out for study in depth, and since still another large-scale study is currently under way, the authors have devoted their attention primarily to the 1.2 million other health workers who fall within the rubric of allied health manpower. This large grouping contains five categories of technicians: x-ray, medical records, occupational and physical therapy, medical, and dental; and three large categories of assistants: licensed practical nurses, nurse's aides, and psychiatric aides.

It may be helpful to set out briefly the major characteristics of these allied health workers and the major trends that can be identified with respect to their recruitment and utilization. This will provide a solid base from which to explore alternative public policies for more effectively utilizing this large and important group to provide essential health services for the American people.

As to their characteristics: reference has already been made to their level of education, which ranges from less than elementary-school completion to just short of college graduation. The median level is one year of college. The overwhelming majority, about 4 out of 5, are women, who tend to be composed of two sub-groups: those in their late teens, and those in their late thirties or above. The fact that about 40 percent of all women workers in the field are under 35 years of age suggests that many health workers tend to drop out of the labor force after a few years and start to raise families. Many come back, part time or full time, but usually not until their youngest child is in school.

Reliance on large numbers of modestly educated young female workers who remain at work for a limited number of years helps to explain the proliferation of training programs, particularly those which present short courses. Since health training below the professional level is only slowly being integrated into the formal educational system—that is, in vocational and comprehensive high schools and in junior and senior colleges—hospitals and other large medical institutions have had to train their own recruits. Much of the training has been short and of indifferent quality—just enough to enable the newcomer to carry out certain limited functions under strict supervision.

The heavy reliance of the health services industry on female labor also helps to explain the relatively low wage rates that have prevailed and which continue to prevail in most regions of the country. Men stay away from jobs which offer little prospect of income sufficient to support a family at a modest level even after many years of work. And the relatively small number of men in the allied health occupations operates to depress the wage scales.

These tendencies have been compounded by federal and state legislation which excluded hospital employees from the provisions of fair labor standards acts and which further interdicted the unionization of hospital workers. While recent changes have occurred on both fronts, wages and working conditions in the health services industry continue to lag behind the more advanced sectors of the economy.

Despite these shortcomings and lags, the industry was able to expand its work force rapidly during the recent past. Between 1950 and 1965, employees on nonagricultural payrolls increased by one-third—from 45 to 60 million. During the same period, total health manpower increased from 1.5 to 2.8 million, or by 87 percent, that is, two and a half times the rate for the economy as a whole.

Several factors contributed to this growth. First, the last two decades have witnessed rapid increases in the overall proportion of women who are actively engaged in remunerative employment, and the health services industry has been traditionally hospitable to women workers. Moreover, hospitals were able to absorb large numbers of untrained workers and many of the women who sought employment were untrained. Next, hospitals located in the large urban centers found that the only prospect of their securing the large numbers of workers they required to meet their replacement and expansion needs was through abandoning their racially discriminatory practices. The health services industry began to attract ever larger numbers of minority group members. This tendency was reinforced by the thrust of recent federal manpower programs which placed heavy emphasis on health training for minority group members.

There is only one way to read the record. Despite the embryonic state of health planning, despite the inherent difficulties of managing a hospital because of the insistence of the physician on a role in administration, despite the hospitals' need to rely on recruiting and training local people, despite historic low wage structures, despite the large turnover rates characteristic of a young female labor supply—despite these and other difficulties and hurdles, the hospitals and other health institutions have demonstrated a remarkable capacity to attract and retain ever larger numbers of allied health manpower so that today these nonprofessionals account for just under half of all the persons engaged in providing health services to the American people. If the record since the end of World War II can be interpreted in so favorable a light, what ground is there for concern about the future?

There are several untoward factors that cannot be ignored. The cost of medical, primarily hospital, care is rising steeply, and wages and salaries account for about 70 percent of the total. The only prospect of moderating this advance is through methods that could slow the rise in wage costs. The fact that more federal money is flowing into the financing of hospital care through Medicare and Medicaid, together with changes in legislative and administrative practices facilitating unionization, are both likely to operate in the opposite direction. The pressure for wage increases, especially for the lowly paid, will be intensified. So much on the cost side.

Consideration must also be given to the forces that continue to operate on the side of demand. The American public has taken at least halting steps in recent years to broaden the access to health services of the poor and the near poor. New experiments to deliver health services to the ghetto populations are under way. A large-scale expansion of nursing care for the aged is definitely planned. In addition to these pressures to meet the hitherto unmet demands for various types of health care of important groups in the population, the leadership in medicine continues to stress that real progress requires that quality gains go hand in hand with increases in the quantity of services to be provided. With allied health manpower often trained in makeshift programs, with many leaving employment a few years after being trained, with professional barriers to the orderly progression of those who acquire knowledge and experience, licensing requirements, and poor personnel management, the obstacles to quality improvement are as serious, if not more, than those standing in the way of meeting the quantitative manpower goals implicit in an expanding system of health care. It is against this background that the potentialities for public policy must be assessed.

A careful reading of this book suggests that improvements in the recruitment, education and training, and utilization of allied health manpower can come about only through a variety of innovative actions at many different leverage points in the system of medical and health care.

To begin with recruitment. A field which attracts a disproportionate number of women, many of them young, will tend to have the following characteristics: a low wage scale, heavy turnover, excessive training costs, and relatively little accumulation of skill through experience. While some of these characteristics, such as a relatively low wage scale, are attractive to employers, it is not a pure gain especially in an industry which confronts the need for rapid growth. Moreover, if an industry cannot meet competitive wage standards it runs the additional risk of not attracting the quality of workers who can absorb training and experience and readily be promoted.

A few experiments are under way on the East Coast, in the South, and in the West to attract into the civilian health industry former servicemen who were trained for and assigned to medical duties while on active service and who enjoyed their work and would be happy to continue in it if they could foresee a reasonable career ahead. Obvious social and personal gains would follow the building of such bridges. But recruitment is the easier part of the effort. The real challenge is to the hospitals and other health agencies which must open up meaningful career opportunities for those working at the lower levels of the hierarchy.

The pressure of unionization, which is slowly growing, should contribute to the building of bridges between occupational levels. Among the most important demands that workers usually make is an expansion of opportunities to which they have access. Currently, the availability of federal training funds, particularly MDTA funds, have made it easier for a few progressive unions and employers to design training programs aimed at the eventual promotion of workers from less-skilled to more-skilled jobs.

But obstacles remain to introducing mobility in the health manpower hierarchy for workers who begin at or near the bottom. At each rung of the ladder there can be found one or more organized groups whose principal aim has been to erect barriers aimed at reducing other workers' access. In most instances they have succeeded in gaining the approval of the state training authorities for their conditions and often they have further protected themselves by having their requirements approved by one of the principal health organizations, such as the American Medical Association or the American Hospital Association. Under these conditions they are in a powerful position to fend off encroachment.

It will require the cooperative efforts of many different groups to reduce barriers that have no justification other than to protect the position of those already ensconced. The demand for health care continues apace, and if the only foreseeable way of meeting this demand is through the rapid expansion of allied health manpower, the preconditions for some easing of restrictive arrangements may exist if hospitals and nursing homes join together with trade unions, medical societies, state licensing boards, and consumer groups to rewrite the laws and administrative practices, and if they move simultaneously and energetically to develop effective training and promotion policies which will open multiple career lines. It can be done, but it surely will not be easy.

A second major thrust must be to improve the education and training of allied health manpower. In recent years a beginning has been made to move beyond the confines of the individual hospital which in the past was the principal and sometimes the sole trainer of health personnel and to expand training through vocational education in high school, in junior colleges, and in the newly established schools of allied health. These are important steps, and when these extensions have stressed a common core of much of the training, they have contributed to the eventual mobility of the manpower pool. Moreover, the transfer of much of the responsibility for didactic health training to the educational system should lead to a strengthening of the curriculum.

But once again we must beware of the difficulties that lie along this route. In the past most state departments of health and education have had little to do with one another. Yet this new approach will require that they work in close harmony if the program is to succeed. Moreover, many young people who enter junior or senior college are likely to be pressed to take a broad liberal arts program together with their vocational or technical courses. In any case the collegiate environment encourages them to become more interested in acquiring a degree than in a salable skill. Finally, many, if not most, hospitals provide training free of charge and some even pay their trainees a modest sum, whereas in most junior and senior colleges students must pay tuition and fees. In shifting more and more training from the hospital to the educational system, care must be taken not to freeze out the many young people from low-income homes which have provided in the past, and must be expected to provide in the future, a significant proportion of all recruits to the health services industry. Liberal scholarship programs and expanded work–study arrangements might compensate for these untoward concomitants of a shift in the training sector.

In recent years the federal government, through the Allied Health Professions Personnel Training Act of 1966, has sought to contribute to the expansion of allied health manpower through appropriating modest sums for expanding and improving training facilities, for the training of faculty, and for the support of experimental programs aimed at increasing the quantity and improving the quality of the total training effort. The current level of federal financing for these several purposes is about $14 million per annum. It is never safe to guess the future actions of Congress, but it appears unlikely that federal appropriations will be significantly increased in the foreseeable future when consideration is given to the present cautionary attitude toward all research and development spending, the priority position of physicians and nurses in commanding financial support, and the fact that in allied health manpower there are such large numbers of persons that any effort to single out their education for federal support would carry an implicit move to subsidize junior and senior college education on a large scale. Until Congress makes a major move in this direction, it is questionable whether it will take but modest additional steps to support directly the education and training of allied health manpower.

The federal effort consists of more than this single act. At its last session Congress undertook a major national commitment to increase federal appropriations for vocational education. And while the health occupations account for a small percentage of all training, circa 5 percent, it is likely that they will expand rapidly.

Attention must also be directed to the Manpower Development and Training Act, which was extended by overwhelming bipartisan support at the last session of Congress. Expenditure levels under this Act are at about half a billion dollars annually and about 20 percent of all training is in the health occupations. Clearly this is a sizable contribution.

Reference has been made to the constant and large-scale training in the health professions provided by the Armed Services and the prospects that exist if the civilian sector can introduce reforms which will enable it to use the ex-servicemen who have been trained and who served in medical assignments.

A comprehensive review of the potential contribution of the federal government would also include reference to the experimental community health centers under the Office of Economic Opportunity, the Regional Programs for Heart, Stroke, and Cancer, and the institutional and program efforts in mental health, vocational rehabilitation, public health, and care for veterans for which the federal government trains or finances the training of allied health manpower.

Nevertheless, the locus for action under our present distribution of responsibilities lies with state and local governments, which continue to have primary responsibility for the financing of education at the secondary and post-secondary levels. Whether the communities of the United States will be able to secure the numbers and the quality of allied health manpower they need to meet the steadily expanding demands for medical and health care will depend primarily on the capabilities of the existing health institutions to continue to train their own people, and whether state and local governments are willing and able to make public funds available to broaden and strengthen the training structure by bringing it increasingly under the rubric of the public educational system.

However, effective recruitment and utilization, as distinct from training, will continue to depend on the nongovernmental sector. The health services industry will be able to attract and retain the numbers and quality of allied health manpower that it will need to meet its expanding requirements only if the several leadership groups—hospitals, trade unions, professional organizations, consumers—recognize the need for change. No industry can respond effectively to the market unless it can attract the resources it requires.

The health services industry will continue to require large numbers of additional workers below the professional level. The challenge it faces is to modernize and rationalize its career structure so that the numbers it will require will be attracted into training and into employment.

ELI GINZBERG

New York City
January, 1969

Acknowledgments

OUR TASKS in gathering and analyzing the data for this book were made less formidable than they might have been for a variety of reasons. First, we were initially guided into this area by Professor Eli Ginzberg, who at all stages gave us the benefit of his vast knowledge of this field. Second, our colleagues in the Conservation of Human Resources Project were always available for soundings of our ideas. Particularly helpful were Professor Dale L. Hiestand and Mrs. Miriam Ostow, who read the entire manuscript and made many constructive comments on it. Third, we received the wholehearted cooperation of dozens of people in the health field—hospital administrators, comptrollers, department heads, and health personnel of all kinds. Last, many government agencies, including Air Force hospitals and Army medical training centers gave us invaluable help and insights.

For the technical aspects of converting illegible script to type and for excellent coordination services we have Mrs. Sylvia Leef to thank. Mrs. Ruth Szold Ginzberg gave us the benefit of her editorial skills. We wish also to acknowledge the very valuable services of Miss Joan McQuary of Columbia University Press.

Since we are jointly responsible for the output, we assume joint responsibility for all errors.

H. I. G.
C. A. B.

Contents

Allied Health Manpower:
Trends and Prospects

CHAPTER 1

Manpower Dynamics of
the Health Services Industry

ONE SELDOM READS alarming reports concerning manpower short-ages in the automobile industry, the shoe industry, the machine tool industry, the textile industry, or the building maintenance industry. Discussions of labor supply in these industries turn on a few fac-tors: wages, working conditions (including automation), and unionization. No one has warned us that in x number of years there will not be enough automobile workers to satisfy the economy's de-mand for cars, or what is worse, that there are not enough auto workers right now to meet the demand for motor vehicles.

Not so in the health services industry. The volume of reports on the present and impending shortages of manpower in this sector has reached torrential proportions. Why here and not elsewhere in the labor force? Are manpower problems in the health field different from those in other fields? If so, what are the differences? If not, why the ubiquitous concern?

The present chapter seeks answers to these questions by way of an examination of some basic economic factors associated with the provision of health services in our economy.

Manpower As an Input

In conventional terms, the output of goods and/or services is accomplished by the entrepreneurially managed interaction of labor and capital. It is the unique function of the entrepreneur (public or private) to maximize output with the resources at his command or, alternatively, to produce a given output at the least cost. He arrives at either of these goals by a judicious combination of the inputs, taking account of prices of the input factors, prices of possible substitute factors, as well as their respective productivities (at the margin). Variations in prices and productivities of input factors lead to the entrepreneur's combining them in different proportions (technological coefficients). The nature of the various inputs (e.g., the degree to which they are divisible) determines the limits within which they may substitute for each other. Thus, labor inputs may, to some degree, be substituted for capital and vice versa, and units of unskilled labor may, to some extent, be substituted for units of skilled labor to produce a given output. The entrepreneur must also take cognizance of the fact that the use of certain types of inputs necessitates the use of complementary inputs, as, for example, when the purchase of a car requires the purchase of gasoline or when the purchase (or lease) of any X-ray machine by a hospital requires the hiring of X-ray technicians.

How does this simplified model of the productive process apply to the output of medical goods and services? A word first about the nature of medical output. In terms of our national income accounts, the total value of all medical goods and services produced in 1965 was $40.8 billion, or approximately 6 percent of the gross national product. Roughly 75 percent of this medical output is accounted for by private spending and 25 percent by government (all levels) spending. Of the $28.1 billion spent in the private sector by consumers, 79 percent went to purchase services, e.g., hospital care, physicians' and dentists' services, nursing-home care, and insurance; the remaining 21 percent purchased goods, e.g., drugs and sundries, eyeglasses, and medical appliances.[1] (In terms of money flow, it might be pointed out here that about half of the cost of medical goods and services is paid directly by the consumer to the vendor and the other half is provided indirectly through so-called third parties.) The demand for medical care then is predominantly a demand for personal services. The latter, for the most part, are provided directly by people (physicians, dentists, nurses) rather than indirectly by machines, and it is for this reason that the medical care industry is sometimes characterized as "labor intensive." Of course, services cannot be provided in a vacuum and, to a large degree, the capital equipment in physicians' and dentists' offices, in clinics, and most importantly that represented by hospital plant and equipment, must be included with the input factors. But even in hospitals, wages and salaries constitute between 60 and 70 percent of total expenses.

In the broader context of industrial classification, medical services come under the services sector of the economy, if one views the entire output of the economy as consisting of the services plus the goods sectors. It should be noted in passing that the services sector is now the larger of the two in terms of manpower employed. For some analytical purposes, it is useful to divide the output of both the goods and services sectors into producer and consumer segments—that is to say, by major type of purchaser. Thus, medical services by and large may be treated under the consumer segment of the services sector in as much as most such services are purchased by (or for) the consumer as final demand. Medical services provided by government, as in the Armed Services, Veterans Administration, and Public Health Work, are also, for the most part, services to consumers. Technically, medical services provided on

---

[1] Ruth S. Hanft, "National Health Expenditures, 1950–65," *Social Security Bulletin,* Vol. 30 (February 1967) Table 1, p. 5.

the job to employees by their employers might be considered a producer service—that is, the medical personnel involved are selling their services to producers (the purchaser) rather than to consumers, and the function of these services is to help maximize the workers' output. In any event, the quantity of such industrial medical services provided and the numbers of medical personnel involved are relatively small.

One must be careful, however, not to apply generalizations to medical services concerning manpower which are derived from studies of services as a whole, since there are many important differences between the demand for medical services and the demand, let us say, for haircuts, movies, maintenance workers, management consultants, and so on.[2] To take one instance here: the fact that illness for an individual (chronic diseases excepted) is unpredictable implies that individual demand for medical services is bound to be irregular unlike the individual's demand for transportation services to his place of employment, for example. Furthermore, since neither the amounts nor the types of illness are predictable (they are more predictable, of course, for large groups than for the individual) the staffing patterns in hospitals contain a large element of inflexibility: many contingencies must be prepared for.

A characteristic often overlooked with respect to the demand for medical services is that there is a certain expandability about it. As the community becomes more aware, for instance, of the nature and manifestations of mental illness, the demand for psychological and psychiatric services grows and usually at a greater rate than the supply of the types and amounts of health manpower needed to provide them. It would be difficult to conceive of any other goods or services which share this characteristic to anywhere near the

[2] Herbert E. Klarman, *The Economics of Health* (New York, Columbia University Press, 1965), pp. 10–19.

same degree. Moreover, as Rene Dubos has pointed out: "It is
. . . the common experience that as some diseases are rooted out,
others spring up to take their place." [3] Not only do some micro-
organisms develop resistance to drugs to which they originally suc-
cumbed, but the environmental changes of a complex economy
generate a host of new diseases with which the populace must con-
tinuously contend. These unique characteristics of the demand for
medical services have important implications for manpower analysis. They imply, for example, that it is much more difficult to talk
about satiation of demand for medical goods and services than it
might be for food, clothing, and shelter in conventional demand
analysis. And perhaps the greatest difficulty in this area is the definition and evaluation of the end product itself—health.

In the context of our simplified production model, the mix of
input factors (technical production coefficients) is heavily weighted
toward labor rather than toward capital (excluding, for the mo-
ment, the fixed plant), but this is by no means a static situation.
Machines and computers are increasingly being utilized to perform
functions previously performed only by physicians, biochemists,
medical technologists, and the like.[4] By contrast, the output of the
goods side of medicine (e.g., drugs) is highly mechanized (capital
intensive) with one tableting machine capable of producing hundreds of thousands of (say) aspirin tablets per day.

So much, therefore, for a generalized view of the production
function in medicine. The next step is to concretize the model by
bringing into the picture such factors as the form and scale of the
enterprise (production) units.

---

[3] Rene Dubos, "Man Meets His Environment," in *Health and Nutrition,* Vol.
VI of the series *Science, Technology, and Development,* U.S. papers prepared for
the United Nations Conference on the Application of Science and Technology for
the Benefit of the Less Developed Nations (Washington [date?]), p. 3.

[4] "Technology and Manpower in the Health Service Industry, 1965–75," *Manpower Research Bulletin No. 14* (Washington, Dept. of Labor, May 1967), ch. 2.

Form of Enterprise in Medicine

In sharp contrast to the rapid scientific developments in biomedical science, organizational forms in medicine are slow to change. The long established procedure for an individual to follow when he perceives a need (demand) for medical attention is to pay a visit to the office (enterprise site) of a physician or dentist. Technically, this is analogous to going to the grocery store when one has a need (demand) for a loaf of bread or, since a service is involved, to going to a barber shop for a haircut. One great procedural change within the last century is that formerly the physician paid a visit to the home of the patient. Another is that there has been an increasing use of hospitals both by inpatients and outpatients. A third is the increasing use of such facilities as nursing homes and public health clinics.

In the vast majority of cases, the physician or dentist or podiatrist in private practice will be a solo practitioner or, in accounting terminology, his business is considered to be a sole proprietorship as distinct from a partnership or corporation. His function in an economic sense is analogous to that of the entrepreneur in our simple model. In many respects his behavior is similar to other self-employed persons; in some it is somewhat different. To some extent he desires and is able to trade off income for leisure. As a well-trained professional he also desires to render medical services of a high quality while retaining a great degree of personal freedom. And in the Hippocratic tradition, he, more than other types of self-employed professionals, will render care at lower or no price to those who cannot afford to pay for his services. (Sliding fee scales are partly compensatory here.) It is important to note at this point that there is a slow but perceptible trend away from private practice. In 1950, 72.1 percent of all physicians were reported as being engaged in private practice (fee-for-service and physician billing were the major criteria). By 1966, the ratio had decreased to 61 percent.[5] The remaining numbers of physicians were divided among full-time hospital staff, interns and residents, full-time teaching, or retired. Those physicians who opt for the not-for-profit sector in general are substituting, for higher income and independence, such things as desire to teach, to practice better medicine, to do full-time research, or some combination of these. Thus the simple model of the maximizing entrepreneur must, in the case of medicine, be appropriately qualified.

The data in Table 1.1 show the types of enterprise forms in medical establishments as of 1964. In the case of physicians and surgeons, 91 percent of the offices were solo practitioners and 9 percent were partnerships,[6] and for dentists and dental surgeons, 98 percent of the establishments were operated as sole proprietorships. It is interesting to note that whereas the partnership arrangement accounted for 9 percent of the total physicians' offices, it accounted for 28 percent of total receipts. This may be attributed to several factors: more practitioners per office, more supporting personnel, more services rendered, and greater productivity per physician. It is also interesting to note that the partnership arrangement is found less frequently in the dental field. Since it is well known that, in general, dentists utilize more ancillary workers in their offices than do physicians, this may lessen the need to derive these advantages via the partnership form. The main point of the table however is clear; the predominant enterprise form in private medical establishments of all types is the sole proprietorship—95 percent of the total in 1964.

Now, the nature of the service the physician renders consists of

[5] "Distribution of Physicians, Hospitals, and Hospital Beds in the U.S." (Chicago, American Medical Association, 1966), Table A, pp. 4–5.

[6] The 1964 data do not show corporate forms separately for physicians and surgeons; in 1961–68 these Internal Revenue Service reports listed some 75 corporations of the then 154,429 offices of physicians and surgeons with the corporations accounting for approximately 1 percent of total receipts.

Table 1.1

Enterprise Forms in Medicine, 1964 *

	Total		Physicians and Surgeons		Dentists and Dental Surgeons		Other Medical and Health Services †	
	Number	Percent	Number	Percent	Number	Percent	Number	Percent
Businesses	424,250	100	169,055	100	87,000	100	168,000	100
Single Proprietorship	402,163	95	153,755	91	85,445	98	162,963	97
Partnership	22,087	5	15,300	9	1,595	2	5,192	3
Business Receipts (in thousands)	$12,436,205	100	$7,604,678	100	$2,641,692	100	$2,189,835	100
Single Proprietorship	$9,725,182	78	$5,475,265	72	$2,513,972	95	$1,735,945	79
Partnership	$2,711,023	22	$2,129,413	28	$127,720	5	$453,890	21

* Excluding hospitals and clinics.
† Including offices of osteopathic physicians, chiropractors, optometrists, podiatrists, and medical and dental laboratories.
Source: Adapted from Treasury Dept. Internal Revenue Service, "U.S. Business Tax Returns, Statistics of Income . . . 1964."

diagnosing the patient's illness by means of visual, instrumental, or laboratory tests and prescribing appropriate therapy which may consist merely of rest, of some form of self-treatment, of a drug which the patient usually purchases at a pharmacy or one which may be injected immediately by the physician, or of a recommendation for hospitalization. (The latter, in turn, involves another input-output cycle which shall be dealt with subsequently.)

Like the grocer, the barber, and the case in most small businesses, the entrepreneur and the labor input are embodied in one person—the solo practitioner. In the present illustration, there were few opportunities to substitute capital for labor—the instruments were usually complements rather than substitutes for the physician's labor and little opportunity to substitute less-skilled labor units for the highly skilled one. Depending on the physician's skill and on the complexity of illnesses presented to him, the number of patients seen per day (his output) was generally a function of the number of hours he chose to work and of the income level he desired to achieve. Some physicians, notably those beginning to build a practice, may be considered as operating at less than full capacity. All output must have a quantitative as well as a qualitative dimension, the latter, in the present instance, depending on the skill of the physician and on the state of the medical art.

Under the circumstances described, shortages of (medical) labor could become manifest in a number of ways: 1) the individual physician would find it increasingly difficult to treat all the patients who sought (demanded) his services even at the cost of excessively long hours (a partial adjustment is possible here in the reduction of time he allocates to each patient, but this might be achieved at the expense of a reduction in the quality of the output); 2) fees for services may increase due to the pressure of demand on supply (to be meaningful in this context the fees would have to increase at a greater rate than fees or prices of other goods and services); 3) because of point 1 or 2 or both, consumers begin to seek other (less expensive or more accessible or both) forms of treatment or more specifically, other types of practitioners. As Professor Boulding has put it: "Monopolistic restriction of entry under the guise of high professional standards has been so great that it has resulted in the development of a number of subprofessions ranging from the osteopath to the Christian Science Practitioner who undercut the regular medicos in the sickness market." [7] Of course, fees are not the sole factor responsible for the growth of some of these "subprofessions" —religious beliefs, misinformation, and lack of knowledge also play a part.

The Division of Medical Labor

Faced with a demand for his services which he could not completely satisfy, the solo practitioner realized, consciously or not, that if he could increase his productivity (number of patients seen per time period) his income would increase significantly. He was therefore induced to find ways and means of conserving his scarce labor power. One of the first techniques used to accomplish this goal has already been mentioned—gradually and with improvements in transportation, especially with the advent of the motor car, patients began to come to the doctor rather than the other way around. Thus, the physician gained a tremendous increase in time which he could devote to seeing patients, with a consequent vast increase in productivity. It goes without saying that from society's point of view, this time gain by the physician must be offset by the possible time loss of the patients who now wait in the office.

To a lesser extent, the physician could gain productivity increases by the use of better and more types of capital equipment such as X-ray machines, fluoroscopes, and the like, but in most

[7] Kenneth E. Boulding, "An Economist's View of the Manpower Concept," in National Manpower Council, *Policy for Utilization of Scientific and Professional Manpower* (New York, Columbia University Press, 1954), p. 23.

cases the types of equipment that could effect real labor savings are uneconomical for the solo practitioner.

But these adjustments to the shortage of medical labor time, important as they were and still are, were not sufficient—the number of patients waiting to be seen continued to increase or, to state it otherwise, the demand for the output of the physician continued to outpace the labor which he could apply to the production process. The only other avenue for increasing his productivity lay in a careful analysis of the functions he actually performed in producing medical services with the aim of so dividing them that others (units of lower skilled and presumably therefore more available) could perform them with equal, and in time, perhaps even greater skill. The professional nurse was seen by the physician as the person who could, because of her knowledge, undertake the routine functions involved in the provision of medical services and, in this way, further conserve the scarce labor time of the physician. The nurse could take temperatures, pulse rates and blood pressures, do routine height and weight measurements, prepare patients for medical or surgical procedures, perform urine and blood tests, and where legally permissible give injections.

For the majority of solo (general) practitioners, this is as far as the division of labor has progressed. Currently these nursing functions are increasingly being performed by even less-skilled units of medical labor, namely the so-called medical assistants.

An additional area for labor saving by the solo practitioner occurs in the use of independent laboratories for the performance of certain biochemical tests or for the taking of X-rays. To some extent, these are tests that the physician and/or his assistant previously performed in-house, as it were, and therefore result in labor saving, but probably to a larger extent, these are tests that require specialized skills and equipment which are either not available in the office or which, in the case of equipment, not economical for the individual physician to purchase due to its relatively infrequent use.

For the sake of completeness, one should mention that certain book-keeping and other office functions are now also being contracted-out with some time-saving possibly resulting.

Two other techniques for conserving the labor time of the physician should be mentioned—so-called group practice and the use of offices in hospitals. In the case of group practice a change in organization and in enterprise form is involved. While group arrangements vary, they essentially involve the sharing of an office or clinic facility by several physicians. This joint use of space, equipment, and clerical personnel should result in greater efficiency (hence lower costs). In theory, the availability of different medical specialists ought also to result in a saving of the patient's time as well as in the receipt of a higher quality of medical care through the close interaction of the several physicians. This type of production facility is preferred by some of the prepayment plans (such as Health Insurance Plan of New York or Kaiser Permanente in California) but may exist under private fee-for-service practice as well. Precisely how much medical labor time is actually conserved by this technique and whether, in fact, a higher quality of output results remain open questions.

The use of the hospital as a site for seeing patients privately is generally a type of fringe benefit given by the hospital to physicians who are on the full-time teaching, clinical, or research staffs as a means of supplementing their incomes. This is therefore not a choice which is open to the average private practitioner.

It would appear, then, that the typically small size of the firm where medical services are largely provided imposes a major constraint on the extent to which the advantages of division of labor and other economies of scale may be realized. The same situation, of course, applies in law, accounting, and in many other professions.

It is plausible to argue that the employment of sub-, non-, or para-professional personnel is *ipso facto* a measure of shortage.

Until the pressure of demand on independent professionals is extremely great, technicians are not likely to be utilized. In fact legislation, framed largely by professional organizations, prevents persons of less skill from performing certain functions which are in the domain of professionals. The income incentive which is inherent in a fee-for-service arrangement operates to inhibit the loss of income-producing services.

It is only when the demand is so great as to outweigh the loss of services that professionals accede to the technicians performance of certain functions first on a *de facto* then a *de jure* basis. In the case of medical care progressively more functions previously considered a monopoly of the physician are being performed by technicians, such as the nurse, the laboratory technician, the X-ray technician, the therapist, and so on. Physicians' incomes have not declined in the process and, in fact, may have increased relatively due to the greater volume of services now possible. Certainly all of the available studies indicate that dentists who utilize auxiliary workers enjoy higher incomes than those who do not.

This does not imply that there are no other reasons for the introduction of technicians. Changes in technology such as for example, the use of radioisotopes, have necessitated the training of entirely new types of technicians, apart from any other factors.

Hospital-Produced Medical Services

As was mentioned earlier, one of the outputs of the individual physician may consist of advising the patient to be hospitalized. Alternatively, the patient may arrive at a hospital by way of an accident or through a visit to the hospital clinic. In any event, the situation analytically is the equivalent of a local auto mechanic indicating to the automobile owner that the repairs required are of such a nature that they cannot be performed at the local garage for reasons of lack of skill, equipment, or storage space and can therefore only be performed at a much larger repair establishment. So with hospitalization.

The hospital then represents a larger scale of enterprise unit than that of the physician's office but functionally it is similar—it is a site where an output (medical service) is sought by a consumer and where inputs in the form of medical manpower and medical plant and equipment are combined to produce same. The hospital differs from the individual office not only in terms of scale but usually in enterprise form. In place of private ownership, most hospitals are of the voluntary nonprofit variety or are government owned, and managerial functions and responsibilities are usually diffused among groups such as administrators, medical chiefs, and boards of trustees. Since the respective goals of these groups may not be similar, the model even of the profit maximizing corporation with a centralized management is inapplicable.

The more significant difference between the hospital and the physician's office lies in the scale of operation. As in any large-scale enterprise, it is easier to take advantage of the efficiencies afforded by the division of labor and specialization. Equipment that is not economical or practicable in the private office becomes feasible in the hospital; medical and surgical procedures which cannot be performed in the office are eminently more suited to the hospital; bed care with intensive medical treatments, and with its associated requirements of laundry and food, is only possible in a hospital or similar institutional setting. On the manpower side, the division of labor is now free to proceed to the limits allowed by the extent of the market: the nursing function, for example, may now be parceled out among RN's, LPN's (licensed practical nurses), and nurse's aides with the result that many more patients may be cared for than was possible when, as in the physician's office or in the hospitals of yesterday, the registered professional nurses alone took temperatures, changed linen, and scrubbed floors.

On the negative side, the hospital, as is true of other large-scale enterprises, may suffer from inefficiencies such as improper internal communication, bureaucratic red tape, inflexibility, and the like. But there is no single hospital the size of General Motors or of the Metropolitan Life Insurance Company so that the managerial inefficiencies which are generally attributable to very large size of firm and to the proliferation and geographic distribution of subsidiary units do not exist to the same degree. A possible exception may be the large number of hospitals under federal, state, county, and municipal control, but no generalizations should be made. In all probability, a great deal of decentralized responsibility acts as an offset to possible centrally generated inefficiency. Moreover, as a recent report from the Army Surgeon General's office pointed out: "It is recognized that a centrally controlled and funded group of Army hospitals, uniformly equipped and staffed, will inevitably exhibit certain cost advantages over a group of individually operated civilian hospitals." [8]

In short, the hospital is in a position to avail itself, to a far greater extent than smaller productive units, of the economies of scale. Undoubtedly the efficiency with which hospitals supply medical services varies with their size (measured by beds or any other suitable index), their basic type (i.e., general, psychiatric, etc.), their geographic location, as well as with the quality of administrative, medical, and other personnel.

It should be noted that to a rapidly growing extent, hospitals are also providing medical services to persons who do not require bed care. These services are known as outpatient visits (emergency or clinic) and, in terms of our organizational framework, are intermediary between the office visit and hospitalization. Thus an organizational continuum exists for the provision of medical services consisting of the individual (or group) physician's office, the outpa-

---

[8] "A Decade of Change in U.S. Hospitals, 1953–63," prepared by Review and Analysis Division, Office of the Comptroller, Office of the Surgeon General (Washington, Dept. of the Army, May 1965), pp. 22–23.

tient clinic of the hospital, and the hospital itself. Increasingly, the locus of medical services is shifting away from the first group and toward the latter two. Physicians' visits per person per annum, for instance, increased by 80 percent from 1930 to 1964 (2.5 to 4.5), while during the same period, annual hospital admissions rose by 160 percent—twice the rate. To take a more recent period, whereas our population increased by 36 percent from 1947 to 1966, admissions to hospitals rose by 64 percent and outpatient visits increased by 247 percent.[9]

Other facilities, such as nursing homes offering skilled care and extended care units of one kind or another, may be considered as offshoots of the hospital and represent the operation of the division of labor principle as applied to facilities as well as to personnel. (However, those facilities which offer primarily residential or "custodial" care may, with good reason, be viewed as offshoots of the home rather than the hospital.)

The Quantity and Quality of Health Manpower

In concrete terms, the demand for medical services took the form of "more than 844 million visits to physicians, 294 million dental appointments, and more than 23 million admissions or discharges from general hospitals in 1964. That is, on the average, each person in the United States saw a physician 4.5 times and a dentist 1.6 times and about 128 people in every 1,000 were admitted to and discharged from a general hospital." In addition, there were 125 million outpatient visits to hospitals in the same year.[10] The quantity of medical services provided by nursing homes and related facilities can only be estimated by such parameters as 23,000 facili-

[9] "Health Manpower Perspective: 1967," *Public Health Service Publication No. 1667* (Washington, 1967), p. 5; *Hospitals: Journal of the American Hospital Association,* Vol. 41, Part 2, *Guide Issue* (August 1, 1967), p. 445.

[10] Forrest E. Lindner, "The Health of the American People," *Scientific American,* Vol. 214, No. 6 (June 1966), p. 25 (reprint).

ties with about 593,000 beds, annual expenditures currently (public and private) approaching the $1 billion level, and catering to over 500,000 "residents." [11]

In broader terms, the quantity of manpower required to produce these medical services in 1964 was approximately 4 million, representing about 5.7 percent of the employed civilian labor force and 6.1 percent of nonagricultural employment.[12]

The U.S. Public Health Service distinguishes between the health field (the broader view) and the health services industry (a narrower view). The health services industry employed 2.6 million people as of the 1960 census, but with the addition of about .5 million people, as for example, 70 percent of all veterinarians and 93 percent of all pharmacists who are presently excluded from this category, plus government (all levels), health personnel (military and nonmilitary), and those employed in the manufacture and distribution of medical goods, the total probably exceeds 4 million. Even with the restricted health services industry definition, medical employment ranked third among major sectors and industries in the United States in 1960; with the broader definition they would undoubtedly rank first or second. Table 1.2 provides perspectives in terms of time as well as in terms of the relation to the labor force of health manpower employment. In absolute numbers, while the total labor force grew by some 74 percent and the nonagricultural labor force by 100 percent between 1920 and 1960, employment in the health services rose by approximately 740 percent. In relative

[11] *Hospitals,* Vol. 39, Part 2, *Guide Issue* (August 1965), p. 438; "Nursing Homes and Related Facilities Fact Book," *Public Health Service Publication No. 930-F-4* (February 1963), p. 5; "Nursing Homes and Related Facilities" (Washington, Dept. of Labor, Wage and Hours and Public Contracts Division, January 1966), estimates from data on pp. 12 and 14; and "Employees in Nursing and Personal Care Homes, United States: May–June 1964," National Center for Health Statistics, Series 12, No. 5 (Washington, Public Health Service), p. 3.

[12] "Manpower in the 1960s," *Health Manpower Source Book,* Section 18 (Washington, Dept. of Health, Education, and Welfare, 1964), p. 1; *Economic Report of the President,* 89C1, January 1965, Table B-21, p. 214.

terms, whereas health services employment constituted about 1 percent of the nonagricultural labor force in 1920, forty years later this ratio had increased to about 5 percent and, as was estimated above, to 6.1 percent by 1964. These data reflect, in part, the extent to which the demand for medical services has affected the total health manpower supply as well as its relative importance in the overall distribution of employment.

Table 1.2

Employment in Health Services, 1920–1960

	1920	*1940*	*1950*	*1960*
Total Labor Force (millions)	40.31	53.3	60.1	70.0
Employment in Nonagricultural sector	27.1	32.4	45.2	54.2
Employment in Health Services sector	.31	1.0	1.6	2.6
Health Services as percent of total labor force	*.8*	*1.9*	*2.7*	*3.7*
Health Services as percent of nonagricultural sector	*1.1*	*3.1*	*3.5*	*4.8*

Source: "Historical Statistics of the United States," U.S. Census; U.S. Depts. of Labor and Health, Education, and Welfare.

Focusing on the 1965 data, we may note that physicians, dentists, and others at the doctoral level, a group that might be termed the autonomous health professionals, or the health manpower core, totaled 425,000 (it is the core personnel who usually provide the initial directives to other personnel). Using a 2.6 million health manpower base we find that about 18 percent, or 1 out of every 6 medical personnel, were part of the "core." Alternatively 5 out of 6 are found in other than the "core" operations, an indication of the extent to which allied health manpower are involved in the provision of health services (see Table 2.1).

Due to the rather lengthy production (training) process for the core personnel—ranging from four to ten years or more of post-secondary-school education, the supply of this type of manpower is of necessity not very responsive to short-run demands. On the other hand, many of the noncore personnel may be trained in much shorter periods—as little as one month for nurse's aides, or about one year of post-secondary education for medical and dental assistants.

A case in point here is the recent action of New York City health officials in hiring 100 ward clerks to alleviate an acute shortage of registered nurses in municipal hospitals. This is an illustration of one type of adjustment to health manpower shortages—the utilization of less-trained personnel to perform some of the functions that more highly trained personnel had been performing and thus to allow the latter to specialize in areas which require their special skills. Of course, there are limits to this type of substitution of less-trained for more-trained workers, but it appears that in the medical area these limits have not yet been approached.

It has been estimated, for instance, that up to 40 percent of registered nurses' time is taken up with what are essentially nonnursing duties—clerical, scheduling, routine care, housekeeping, and so on. The realization by hospital administrators that licensed practical nurses can, at lower cost, perform all of these functions has led to relative declines in the proportion of registered nurses employed in hospitals and to corresponding increases in the percentage of licensed practical nurses.

This shorter training period together with changes in the production process for health services that we have treated under the division of labor, plus the newer concepts in the treatment of disease (e.g., health team approach and progressive patient care) have all combined to increase the noncore or allied health personnel at a much greater rate than the core (see Chapter 2). As a consequence the whole nature of the medical input mix is undergoing rapid change.

Dr. Lowell T. Coggeshall, an eminent medical educator, put it this way: "The need for persons trained in related health fields to work as members of the team under the leadership and the coordination of the physician is growing even more rapidly than the need for physicians." [13]

The following chapters will attempt to analyze this change in greater detail with the objectives of providing a clearer picture of medical manpower utilization in the United States and of the implications and effects of manpower policies in the health field.

[13] Lowell T. Coggeshall, "Planning for Medical Progress through Education" (Evanston, Ill., Association of American Medical Colleges, April 1965), p. 26.

CHAPTER 2

Allied Health Personnel in
the Health Manpower Spectrum

LIKE ECONOMIC ANALYSES in general, manpower analysis has been applied more to goods than to services output. Within the services sector, again following the mainstream of economists' investigations, relatively little attention has been paid to the health services. It is small wonder then that we do not have a useful body of health manpower studies to turn to and that each investigator needs to start anew with only his own perspectives and purposes for guidance.

In the previous chapter, the attempt was made to trace the path of the division of labor in the production of health services and to suggest the major causal factors involved in the process. The present chapter seeks to extend this analysis by way of a more detailed look at the quantities and qualities of the existing and newly emerging occupations in the "health industry" and to assess their role in the provision of health services. As a prefatory note, it should be pointed out that our primary concern here is with employment which is industry-specific as distinct from that which is occupation-specific. For example, X-ray technician is an industry-specific category in that such a person is employed only or almost completely in the health industry; on the other hand, a bookkeeper is an occupation-specific title—such a person may be employed in a hospital but also in any other firm or industry. Excluded from the following discussion, therefore, are persons such as those engaged in general clerical and maintenance functions. Obviously, such occupations must be included in the analysis of total manpower problems, but the focus here is primarily on the analysis of industry-specific occupations.

Who Are Allied Health Personnel?

Traditionally, and for valid reasons, the lines of authority in medical matters were rather strictly defined and went in one direction—from the physician downward. In a modern hospital setting, with complex administrative, financial, and medical functions, the older relationships have to be modified. Where this is slow to occur, interpersonal problems are aggravated. With a relatively large and diverse medical labor force, the problems of classification become very important.

Occupational titles, which imply and define relationships between one type of worker and another, are generally pejorative and hence chronic bones of contention. Should the term "professional" for instance be arrogated by and for physicians? What about dentists, podiatrists, "professional nurses," psychologists, and hospital administrators? If it is agreed that all of the foregoing are professionals, does this then relegate nutritionists, health economists, and psychiatric social workers to the categories of semi-, sub-, para-, or quasi-professionals? Are the remainder of the health workers then nonprofessionals? Simply to raise these questions is to reveal the shortcomings and pitfalls of much of traditional occupational nomenclature. In view of these problems it is easy to sympathize with one author who stated that: "This older, clinical concept of 'medical and paramedical' should give way to a more realistic one em-

bracing all of the skilled, semi-skilled, and unskilled personnel dealing with the individual and social health of man." [1] But this approach still raises the problem of determining skill levels, is also in-
vidious in nature and, more importantly, by eliminating all boundaries between disciplines, it precludes the benefits to be derived
from a systematic analysis of the health field per se.

On the other hand, there are some authorities for whom the term
"paramedical" is appropriate. Dr. Marcus Kogel, for instance,
writes:

The term paramedical is an expression of the team approach to medical
care. "Para" is a Greek word meaning alongside of. The physician of today needs a large cast of specialized assistants to work alongside him in
order to provide health service that scientific advances have made possible. The President's Commission on the Health Needs of the Nation
defined paramedical workers as persons other than physicians, dentists,
and nurses who are engaged in the investigation, treatment, and preven-
tion of disease and disability and in the promotion of health by virtue
of some special skill. [2]

So defined, paramedical is not and need not be a disparaging
term. However, because it does appear deprecatory to some groups
and since the term has all but been eliminated from current federal
statistics we shall go along with the mainstream and in the present
study use the term "allied health personnel" as a synonym to denote
all of the health occupations below the (autonomous) doctoral
level.

[1] Frederic J. Moore, "Problems of Planning for an Adequate Number of Para-
Medical Personnel," *Hospital Forum,* Vol. 12, No. 2 (November 1961), p. 19.
[2] Marcus D. Kogel, "Problems and Potentialities of Using Paramedical Person-
nel to Insure the Most Effective Utilization of Medical Personnel," in National
Manpower Council, *Policy for Scientific and Professional Manpower* (New York,
Columbia University Press, 1954), p. 102.

A First Pass Over the Data

The primary source of quantitative occupational data is the decennial census of population.[3] In it, the medical industry is divided into two parts: Medical and Other Health Services, Except Hospitals; and Hospitals. For 1960, total employment in these medical fields was approximately 2.6 million, of whom 1.69 million or 65 percent worked in a hospital setting. The basic characteristics within the two divisions are: male–female and salaried–self-employed.

Overall, 70 percent of health workers are women with a ratio of females to males of 2.3 to 1. Within the hospital setting the female–male ratio is 3 to 1, and among the salaried nonhospital group the ratio is 4.7 to 1. The only category wherein males outnumber females is the nonhospital self-employed group (mainly independent professionals) where the ratio of males to females is 2.9 to 1.

The Census classification of the specific occupations (detailed occupation) however, while useful for some purposes, is not as revealing of the characteristics of health manpower as it might be. To illustrate: dietitians and nutritionists, professional nurses, optometrists, osteopaths, pharmacists, physicians and surgeons, and therapists are all listed under the general rubric of "Professional, Technical and Kindred Workers." All told, not more than about a dozen medical occupations are detailed in the Census, whereas the *Health Manpower Source Book* of the Public Health Service lists about forty major health service occupations.

What the Census classification and data do reveal is that there is a far greater proportion of professional, technical, and kindred workers in the health field in contrast to all other industries (45 percent and 12 percent respectively); that a smaller proportion of

[3] Specifically, "Occupations by Industry," P.C. (2) 70, *U.S. Census of Population, 1960*, Table 2, pp. 132–36.

managers, officials, and proprietors work in health compared with all others (3 percent and 13 percent), and that a higher proportion of service workers are in health (31 percent) relative to other industries (12 percent).[4] But these facts are but a starting point for the analysis of health manpower problems.

Identification of and Alternative Classification Scheme for Health Manpower

For the purposes of a more thorough grasp of health manpower problems and for the formulation of policy in this field, more meaningful classification systems are needed. Apart from gross identification and enumeration, a taxonomic framework should also enable us to gauge the impact of economic changes on health manpower, should provide information useful for occupational guidance, and should serve as a guide in the education and training of such manpower.

Preliminary work on identification of health occupations was provided by the *Dictionary of Occupational Titles,* the *Occupational Outlook Handbook,* and the *Health Careers Guidebook*—all published by the U.S. Department of Labor. Additional work in this area has been done by the National Center for Health Statistics of the U.S. Public Health Service.[5]

Allied health personnel may be separated into three components, the first of which has, for legislative purposes, already been termed "allied health professionals"; the second, which we shall term "allied health technicians"; and the third, "allied health assistants." The basic criterion of demarcation in this scheme is that of educational level. The allied health professionals are those who have at-

[4] "Manpower in the 1960s," *Health Manpower Source Book,* Section 18 (Washington, Dept. of Health, Education, and Welfare), Table 4, p. 6.

[5] "What Are the Health Occupations?" Task Force on Health, Education, and Welfare Manpower Requirements and Training Program, Subcommittee on Health Manpower, *Staff Paper No. 3* (Washington, December 29, 1965).

tained a minimum of a baccalaureate degree and who, in some cases, hold master's and doctoral degrees. The health technicians are those who are trained mainly on the vocational school levels. The third segment of this group, the allied health assistants, are all of the other personnel who are employed in the direct or indirect provision of health services and who have attained various educational levels up to and including high-school graduation.

To complete this occupational structure, physicians, osteopaths, dentists, podiatrists, and optometrists fall into a group which we have already termed autonomous or Core Health Professionals (see Chapter 1).

Following is a listing of health manpower by the proposed divisions:

1. *Autonomous Health Professionals*
   Physicians
   Osteopaths
   Dentists
   Podiatrists
   Optometrists
2. *Allied Health Professionals*
   Professional nurses
   Clinical psychologists
   Cytotechnologists
   Dental hygienists
   Dieticians
   Food technologists
   Hospital administrators
   Immunochematologists
   Medical illustrators
   Medical record librarians
   Medical technologists
   Biostatisticians
   Computer programmers
   Health economists
   Manual arts therapists
   Recreation therapists
   Psychometlists
   Mycologists

Nuclear medical technologists
Nutritionists
Occupational therapists
Physical therapists
Rehabilitation counselors
Speech pathologists and
  audiologists
Virologists
X-ray technologists
Pharmacists
Bioengineers
Health administrators
Health educators
Music therapists
Medical social workers

3. *Allied Health Technicians*
  X-ray technicians
  Registered nurses (Associate degree or diploma)
  Medical records technicians
  Occupational therapy assistants
  Medical technicians
  Medical and dental assistants

4. *Allied Health Assistants*
  Licensed practical nurses
  Nurse's aides
  Psychiatric aides

The personnel in Group 1 for example, are characterized by the fact that all have doctoral level degrees and also by the fact that they exercise independent judgment and bear ultimate responsibility for the diagnosis and management of the patient's illness. Those in Group 2 for the most part work under the direction of autonomous or core personnel and may also exercise a great deal of independent judgment. Those in Groups 3 and 4 work almost entirely under directives from the professionals in Groups 1 and 2, and their range of discretionary activity is extremely narrow. As Ray Brown put it, in discussing the changes over time in the provision of health services: "The individual physician remained the decision-maker in the care of the individual patient, but the implementation of his decisions became in large part an organizational affair requiring the participation of many different skills and the utilization of a complex variety of specialized facilities." [6] A grouping of health manpower, which is based primarily on educational level thus also serves to reveal the interdependence of the health occupations as well as the direction of flow of directives from those occupations which have the greatest degree of discretionary decision-making ability with respect to patient care, to those which have the least.

One thing stands out even at this level of the analysis: we can no longer view the provision of health services solely in terms of the traditional triumvirate of physician, dentist, and nurse. As one pathologist puts it: "The physician can perform no better than the personnel upon whom he depends for laboratory examinations, X-ray examinations, radioisotopic studies, ECG studies, and others." [7] Not only can he perform no better, but the modern physician will perform a lot worse, without at least some assistance from the allied health team. As we have already stated, the key to understanding of health services and of health manpower is interdependence. The inability or unwillingness on the part of some segments of the health field to recognize and come to grips with this economic (and scientific) fact of life is one of the root causes of many problems beclouding the medical manpower scene. Walter Mc-Nerney, in a comprehensive study of Michigan hospitals, cited a statement from a 1960 report of the Western Interstate Commission for Higher Education, which is appropos here: "Too often, health manpower has been considered in terms of doctors, dentists, and nurses alone. Too often, the problems of supporting personnel have

---

[6] Ray E. Brown, "Redefinition of the Hospital," in *The Hospital Patient Outside the Hospital*, a report of the 1966 National Forum on Hospital and Health Affairs (Durham, Duke University, Graduate Program in Hospital Administration, 1966).

[7] *Allied Health Professions Personnel Training Act of 1966*, Hears./HR CIFC/-89C2/1966, p. 25.

been completely overlooked or ignored. But it makes no more sense to ignore the need for supporting personnel in the health sciences than it would to recruit an army of all generals and no privates." [8]

Table 2.1 provides recent data on the numbers of persons in some of the more important health occupations grouped by educational levels approximately as outlined above.

These data show some interesting relationships, especially when viewed in a time perspective. First, whereas physicians at the turn of the century constituted over 80 percent of health occupations (the remaining 17 percent were dentists),[9] their ratio has now been reduced to 12 percent. Second, when we add the other doctoral level occupations to physicians, the core or autonomous health professionals, as we have termed them, now represent about 16 percent of total health manpower, which implies further than 84 percent of total health manpower fall into our allied health personnel category. The chart on page 31 shows the long-term trends in the health manpower mix.

The health occupations at the baccalaureate and masters' levels constitute about 12 percent of the total. Perhaps the most revealing facts derived from these data are that almost half (48.4 percent) of all health service workers fall into the one-to-three-year post-high-school group and that approximately one-fifth (21.7 percent) probably have less than a high-school education. Combining the latter two groups, we then find that fully 70 percent of health service workers have three years or less of college training.

Not only do these data show the extent to which the division of labor in medical services has progressed, but they also provide insights into such problems as income distribution, recruitment, and educational and training requirements.

[8] Walter J. McNerney et al., "Hospital and Medical Economics" (Chicago, Hospital Research and Education Trust, 1962), Vol. I.

[9] "Historical Statistics of the United States, Colonial Times to 1957" (Washington, Bureau of the Census, 1960), p. 34.

Table 2.1

Number of Health Service Workers by Level of Training, 1965

Training and Occupation	Number of Persons	
Total	2,416,000	
Doctoral level	425,000	
Physician (M.D. and D.O.) *		288,000
Dentist		93,000
Other		44,000
Baccalaureate level	295,000	
Medical technologist †		32,000
Occupational therapist		8,000
Physical therapist		12,000
Professional nurse (B.S.)		70,000
Speech pathologist, audiologist		13,000
Other		160,000
3 years of college or less	1,171,000	
Diploma nurse		522,000
Dental hygienist ‡		15,000
Medical record librarian §		10,000
X-ray technologist ‖		70,000
Certified laboratory assistant		1,100
Cytotechnologist		3,000
Dental assistant		95,000
Dental laboratory technician		27,000
Inhalation therapist		4,000
Practical nurse		265,000
Other		159,900
Short training	525,000	

* Active.
† Registered (both B.A. and less than B.A.).
‡ Licensed (some B.A., primarily two-year programs).
§ Employed in hospitals.
‖ Both B.A. and less than B.A.
Note: Estimates by Public Health Service on basis of available data from professional organizations.
Source: Adapted from *Allied Health Professions Personnel Training Act of 1966* (HR 13196), Hears./HR CIFC/89C2/1966, p. 9.

It is important not only to identify the various health occupations but also to measure the change over time in their numbers, as both provide indications of the response of supply to demand as well as of the economy's demand for health compared with other-than health manpower. Accordingly, Tables 2.2 and 2.3 present data

Health Manpower, 1900 and 1966

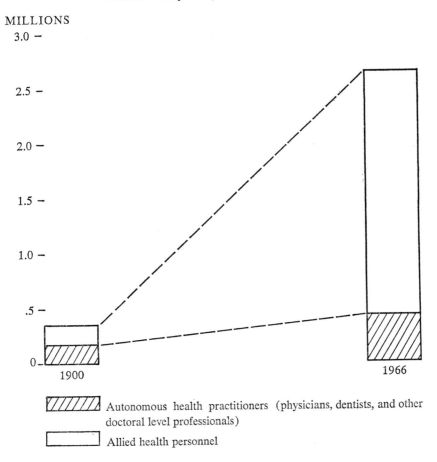

Source: Bureau of the Census and Department of Health, Education, and Welfare.

on total nonagricultural employment and employment in specific health occupations for 1950, 1960, and 1965.

A number of interesting observations may be made with respect to the data in Table 2.2. First, between 1950 and 1960, nonagricul-

Table 2.2

Changes in Nonagricultural and in Health Manpower, 1950–1965

Employment	Nonagricultural (*in millions*)	Health	Ratio (*health as percent of nonagricultural*)
1950	45.2	1.5	3.3
1960	54.2	2.2	4.1
1965	60.4	2.8	4.6
Percent Change			
1950–60	+19.9	+46.7	2.3
1950–65	+33.6	+86.7	2.6
1960–65	+11.4	+26.3	2.4

Source: "Manpower in the 1960s," *Health Manpower Source Book*, Section 18 (Washington, Dept. of Health, Education, and Welfare, 1964), and "Health Resources Statistics, 1965," *Public Health Service Publication No. 1509* (Washington, Dept. of Health, Education, and Welfare, 1965).

tural employment rose by some 20 percent; in the same period, health employment (as defined by the Public Health Service) rose by 46.7 percent, or 2.3 times as fast. Second, for the longer period, 1950 to 1965, while nonagricultural employment increased by 33.6 percent, employment in the health field rose by 86.7 percent, or 2.6 times faster. Third, for the recent five-year period, 1960 to 1965, when nonagricultural employment increased by 11.4 percent, health employment rose by 27.3 percent, or 2.4 times as fast. These relative rates of employment growth may be viewed as one measure of the increasing and persistent demand for health services in recent years. It is important to note too that these data do not reflect the potentially large impact of recent federal legislation in the health field, some of which, like Medicare and Medicaid, operate mainly on the demand side and others, such as the various acts which provide financial assistance to medical students, nurses, and other allied health personnel, attempt to increase the supply of health manpower.

Table 2.3 gives us a view of the change in the numbers of physicians, dentists, and nurses and provides bases for comparison with subsequent data on allied health personnel. As we may note, there is a great similarity in the employment changes for physicians and dentists. In both cases, total population growth between 1950 and 1960 exceeded the increases in the numbers of those professions. Of the three groups, only the nurses increased at a greater rate than did the total population.

Table 2.3

Number of Physicians, Dentists, and Nurses, 1950–1965

	Employment			Percent Change		
	1950	*1960*	*1965*	*1950–60*	*1950–65*	*1960–65*
Physicians (MD and DO)	232,700	274,800	288,000	+18.1	+23.8	+4.8
Dentists	87,200	101,900	105,500	+16.9	+21.0	+3.5
Nurses (RN's)	375,000	504,000	592,000	+34.4	+57.9	+17.5
Total U.S. population (000)	152,271	180,684	193,818	+18.7	+27.3	+7.3

Source: "Manpower in the 1960s," *Health Manpower Source Book,* Section 18 (Washington, Dept. of Health, Education, and Welfare, 1964); House Report 1628, "Allied Health Professions Personnel Training, October 1966"; U.S. Census.

When we turn to allied health occupations specifically (Table 2.4), we find that 22 of the 23 occupations listed exhibited increases in employment between 1950 and 1960.

Using as a norm the 20 percent increase in nonagricultural employment between 1950 and 1960, the data show that in 16 of the 23 occupations (or in 70 percent of those listed) the norm was exceeded. Moreover, if we arbitrarily choose an increase of 100 percent (viz., a doubling of employment and a rate some five times the

Table 2.4

Estimated Employment in Selected Health Occupations

Occupation	Employment			Percent Change		
	1950	1960	1965	1950–60	1960–65	1950–65
Administrator, hospital and other	8,600	12,000		+13		
Dietician, nutritionist	22,000	26,000		+18		
Medical secretary, and office assistant	70,000	80,000		+14		
Medical laboratory technologist-technician	30,000	68,000		+127		
Medical records librarian	4,000	8,000	10,000	+100	+25	+150
Medical records technician	8,000	20,000		+150		
Medical X-ray technologist-technician	30,000	60,000	70,000	+95	+17	+127
Optician, optical laboratory mechanic	19,200	20,300		+6		
Optometrist	17,800	17,300		−3		
Pharmacist	101,000	117,000		+16		

Psychologist, clinical and other health	3,000	8,000		+167		
Rehabilitation counselor	1,500	3,000		+100		
Social worker, medical and psychiatric	6,200	11,700		+89		
Statistician, analyst	2,000	5,000		+150		
Therapist, occupational	2,000	5,000	8,000	+150	+60	+300
Therapist, physical	4,600	9,000	12,000	+96	+33	+161
Therapist, speech and hearing	1,600	6,200	13,000	+288	+97	+713
Dental assistant	55,200	82,500		+50		
Dental hygienist	7,000	12,500		+79	+20	+114
Dental laboratory technician	21,000	25,000		+19		
Practical nurse	137,000	206,000	15,000	+50		
Aide, orderly, attendant	221,000	375,000		+50		
Homemaker, home health aide	500	2,300		+360		

Source: "Manpower in the 1960s," *Health Manpower Source Book*, Section 18 (Washington, Dept. of Health, Education, and Welfare, 1964), Table 8, and House Report 1628, "Allied Health Professions Personnel Training, October 1966," Table 5, p. 11. In cases of discrepancies, data from the House Report were used.

norm) as representing an extremely rapid growth rate over the decade of the 1950s, we find that 9 of the 23 occupations recorded 100 percent or more of employment growth. It might be useful to list these extremely rapidly growing health occupations together with their 1950–60 percentage growth rates:

Medical laboratory technologists and technicians	+127
Medical record librarians	+100
Medical record technicians	+150
Psychologists, clinic and other health workers	+167
Rehabilitation counselors	+100
Statisticians and analyst health personnel	+150
Therapists, occupational	+150
Therapists, speech and hearing	+288
Homemakers, home-health aides	+360

To the above list should be added the two occupations which showed rates of between 95 and 100 percent and which, for all practical purposes, may also be considered to have doubled in employment: physical therapists with a 96 percent increase and medical X-ray technologist-technicians with a 96 percent growth rate.

In part, these very high percentages increases are due to the relatively small absolute numbers involved, but one cannot escape the conclusion that the allied health area as a whole is growing at a significant pace.

A recent publication of the U.S. Department of Labor pointed out that between 1946 and 1961, the number of laboratory procedures per hospital admission rose from 3.19 to 6.36, a 99 percent increase; the number of diagnostic X-ray procedures rose from 1.50 to 4.42, a 195 percent change, and the number of different generic drugs prescribed rose from 4.67 to 7.30, a 56 percent rise. Changes in medical practice such as these involve the heavy use of allied health personnel and explain, in part, the rapid rises shown by the data.[10]

[10] "Technology and Manpower in the Health Services Industry, 1965–1975," *Manpower Research Bulletin No. 14* (Washington, Dept. of Labor, May 1967), Table 7, p. 72.

In the few occupations for which 1960 to 1965 data are available, we find a continuation of the high growth rates of the 1950s. Thus, while total nonagricultural employment rose by about 11 percent between 1960 and 1965, occupational therapists grew by 60 percent, physical therapists by 33 percent, speech and hearing therapists by 97 percent, dental hygienists by 20 percent, medical record librarians by 25 percent, and medical X-ray technologists and technicians by 17 percent.

Taking the longer period, 1950 to 1965, during which time nonagricultural employment grew by about 34 percent, occupational therapists showed a 300 percent increase, physical therapists a 161 percent increase, speech and hearing therapists a remarkable 713 percent increase, dental hygienists a 114 percent rise, medical record librarians a 150 percent growth rate, and medical X-ray technologists grew by 127 percent. Clearly, these medical areas have been absorbing labor at remarkably high and persistent rates.

Functional Classifications

Up to this point the data with which we have been dealing have been arranged descriptively rather than functionally, except for our earlier fourfold classification of health manpower into Autonomous or Core, Professional, Technical, and Assistant categories. In order to relate changes in demand for health services, changes in technology, changes in concepts of disease management, changes in disease types, and general demographic changes to health manpower requirements, a functional approach is necessary—an approach which is rooted in the nature of the services actually rendered by the various health occupations.

One attempt at a functional classification of health occupations is that found in the *Health Manpower Source Book,* section 18, titled "Manpower in the 1960s" (1964), published by the U.S. Public Health Service. In Tables 8 and 9 (pp. 14–15) of that compendium, health manpower is grouped into five major categories: Medical, Dental, Nursing, Environmental, and Research. These divisions enable us to say, for example, that in 1950, 98.7 percent of health manpower were in the three categories of medical, dental, and nursing, and that in 1960, this ratio decreased by 1 percentage point. Thus, while it is a first approximation to an ordering of the universe of health manpower, it is too general to be operationally useful.

In a recent publication, the Public Health Service, Health Manpower Statistics Branch, has moved away from this five-category general scheme to a more detailed classification of health manpower into thirty-five "health fields." [11] In Table 2.5 we have rearranged the thirty-five health fields (which were listed alphabetically in the publication) to reflect the numerical importance of the various groups. (We have used the mean wherever a range of employment was given.) Arranged in this way, the three broadly classified occupations which constituted 97 to 98 percent of total medical manpower in the earlier scheme (i.e., medical, dental, and nursing) now account for only 68.4 percent, a recognition of the existence and importance of other supporting groups in the field.

This tabulation highlights the overwhelming quantitative importance of nursing and related services—still almost 50 percent of total health manpower in 1965 as it was in 1960 and 1950. However, there have been some changes within the nursing occupations between the relative importance of RN's, LPN's and aides. For example, in 1950, professional nurses, i.e., those with Associate or higher degrees represented 51 percent of total nursing personnel; as of 1963, this ratio fell to 46 percent. The ratio of licensed practical nurses remained relatively constant over this period at 19 percent and that of aides rose to 35 from 30 percent in the earlier year.

Doctors and dentists in this table comprise 18.8 percent of total health workers, yielding therefore approximately 81 percent at the

---

[11] "Health Resources Statistics, 1965," *Public Health Service Publication No. 1509* (Washington, Dept. of Health, Education, and Welfare, 1965).

Table 2.5

Estimated Employment in Health Field
by Occupation, 1965

Health Field	Estimated Employment	Percent of Total
All Fields	2,838,800	100.0
1. Nursing and related services	1,409,000	49.6
2. Medicine and osteopathy	305,000	10.7
3. Dentistry and allied services	230,900	8.1
4. Secretarial and office services	200,000	7.1
5. Pharmacy	118,000	4.2
6. Clerical laboratory services	90,000	3.2
7. Radiologic technology	70,000	2.5
8. Basic sciences in health field	44,200	1.6
9. Visual services and eye care	40,400	1.4
10. Medical Records	37,000	1.3
11. Administration of Health Services	34,250	1.2
12. Environmental health	33,750	1.2
13. Dietetic and nutritional service	30,000	1.2
14. Chiropractic and naturopathy	25,000	.90
15. Veterinary medicine	23,700	.80
16. Social work	17,500	.62
17. Health education	16,700	.59
18. Food and drug protective services	16,500	.58
19. Speech pathology, audiology	14,000	.49
20. Physical therapy	12,000	.42
21. Psychology	9,000	.32
22. Library services in health	8,000	.28
23. Podiatry	7,600	.27
24. Biomedical engineering	7,500	.26
25. Misc. hospital services	6,200	.22
26. Occupational therapy	6,000	.21
27. Specialized rehabilitation services	5,600	.20
28. Midwifery	5,000	.18
29. Health information and communication	5,000	.18
30. Vocational rehabilitation and counseling	4,200	.15
31. Orthopedic and prosthetic appliances	3,300	.12
32. Health and vital statistics	1,900	.07
33. Anthropology and sociology	700	.02
34. Economic research in health	500	.02
35. Automatic data processing	300	.01

Source: "Health Resources Statistics," *Public Health Service Publication No. 1509* (Washington, 1965).

less-than-doctoral or allied health levels—a ratio which agrees with one derived earlier from other data. From the standpoint again of educational level we are able to make the statement that 8 out of 10 health workers are at the less-than-doctoral level and, as mentioned earlier, 7 out of 10 health workers or about 70 percent have three years of college training or less.

The fourth highest group in this table is one labeled "Secretarial and Office Services." This group which accounted for about 7 percent of the total, has not been included in previous tabulations and, because it is an occupation-specific rather than an industry-specific classification, it should, for the purposes of this analysis, be treated separately.

The general importance of this tabulation is that it gives a more complete picture of the major health fields and also that it allows one to gain perspective in terms of the quantitative importance of the various occupations and fields. In view of recent trends in health toward progressive patient care, the relatively low ratios to the total of vocational rehabilitation and counseling (.15), specialized rehabilitation services (.20), and occupational therapy (.21) are thrown into sharp relief.

Another recent attempt at a functional classification of health workers is that of Jeffrey Weiss.[12] Weiss, confining his analysis to industry-specific occupations, develops a classification scheme for health manpower wherein jobs are grouped according to two criteria—major technical focus and level of job content. Table 2.6 illustrates the so-called health care job families, into which health manpower is divided together with their relative weights in 1950 and 1960.

The schema marks a step forward in medical manpower classification on two counts: it is functional in nature and it avoids the pejorative connotations of older nomenclature. Comparing some of

---

[12] Jeffrey Weiss, "The Changing Job Structure of Health Manpower" (unpublished dissertation, Harvard University, 1966).

Table 2.6

*Percent Distribution of Manpower
in Health Care Job Families,
1950 and 1960*

Job Family	1950	1960
Patient care		
Medical	18.22	15.37
Dental	6.92	6.56
Mental	2.75	1.20
Nursing	56.42	59.77
Technical and laboratory	13.00	11.86
Administration and planning	2.26	1.89
Data processing	0.92	1.52
Environmental	0.72	0.86
Research	0.78	0.97
Total	100	100

Source: Jeffrey Weiss, "The Changing Job Structure of Health Manpower" (unpublished dissertation, Harvard University, 1966), Table II-B, p. 95.

the ratios of this table (1960) with those of Table 2.5 (1965 data) indicates that while nursing activities still predominate in both, their relative weight in the Weiss scheme is 10 percentage points greater. Weiss's system also yields higher ratios for medical services, 15 percent compared with 10.7 (the disparity would be greater if patient care—mental were added to medical) and in data processing, where the difference is great—.01 percent for the Public Health Service classification and 1.52 for Weiss's. Dentistry receives a lower weight in the Weiss scheme—6.56 as opposed to 8.1 for PHS. These differences, however, are rooted in definitions, not arithmetic, and we have already indicated the general merit of Weiss's typology. Within the context of his own definitions, we would, on intuitive grounds, question the relative declines between 1950 and 1960 recorded in the technical and laboratory focus and in the Health Administration and Planning groups. Perhaps the major conclusion of Weiss's work is his statement that, "While the level of job content of the U.S. has increased over time, the level of job content of health manpower has declined." [13] That is to say, in the "mix" of health occupations, those with low job-content levels have gained relative to those with high and middle levels.

The important analytic proposition behind Weiss's job structure analysis is that the output of health services should be viewed in terms of joint inputs, and further, that there is a greater degree of substitutability among the input factors than has heretofore been acknowledged. But in attempting to correct the implicitly accepted view that health services are produced with fixed coefficients, Weiss strays too close to the proposition that the coefficients are completely variable. He writes in terms of, "the substitution of jobs with relatively lower levels of job content for jobs with relatively higher levels of job content," as if there were in fact a high degree of substitutability involved. The assumptions of continuity and substitutability tend to obscure the real factors operating in the provision of health services in the economy. For example, the physician can do all of the things the nurse can do, and even though the nurse can do many of the things the physician does, there are many things she is not allowed to do either by law or custom. Similar legal or institutional barriers exist throughout the medical manpower field making substitution either impossible or severely limiting its potential, thus giving the character of "noncompeting groups" to the health occupations. Undoubtedly such inflexibility decreases the efficiency of the input factors, but at least the recognition of this situation should be the first step towards improvement. We must also be more mindful of the distinction between substitutes and complements and its implications.[14] In many cases, the "lower level" job-content occupations are complementary to rather than substitutes for the "middle" and "high level" occupations. Lower-level jobs may originate as a result of the process of division of labor in the health services

[13] *Ibid.*, p. 100.   [14] *Ibid.*, p. 77.

area as well as by the introduction of new techniques such as nuclear medicine. The nuclear medical technologist is not a substitute for an older occupation. Finally, Weiss's system emphasizes intra-industry substitutions, but many of the problems of the health industry, especially at the primary level of recruitment and even among those already in the field, have their roots in inter-industry mobility.

An alternative classification system may be developed which is at once more general and more functionally oriented than those which we have considered so far. Such a system stems from a more fundamental view of the major functions of health services, viz., what types of services are demanded by the consumer and provided by the "producers" (i.e., medical personnel, facilities, and equipment). A taxonomic framework based on this approach might be proposed as follows:

Functional Classification of Allied Health Personnel
1. *Diagnostic:* laboratory technicians, X-ray technicians, optometrists, and psychologists.
2. *Therapeutic:* radiological technicians, dental hygienists, and RN's.
3. *Patient Maintenance:* orderlies, attendants, nurse's aides, dieticians, and nutritionists.
4. *Rehabilitative and Supportive:* therapists (occupational, physical, speech, and hearing), prosthetic technicians, social workers (medical and psychiatric), and homemakers.
5. *Administrative:* administrators, medical secretaries and office assistants, medical record librarians, statisticians, and analysts.

Since this outline is aimed primarily at the classification of allied health personnel, the "core" professionals are not included; however, it is clear that most physicians, dentists, podiatrists, and so on would fall into categories 1 and 2, i.e., diagnostic and therapeutic. It is also clear that, as in all classification schemes, there is not only the inevitable overlapping but also the inherent difficulties of marginal classifications. Psychologists, for example, cut across three of the categories: rehabilitative, diagnostic, and curative. Similarly, multipurpose functions may be found with respect to some of the other occupations, but, by and large, this functional differentiation appears to offer a first approximation to a more useful taxonomic framework. Many apparent problems of functional plurality may be resolved when one focuses on the major function of the particular worker.

Several important advantages accrue from this kind of functional classification. In the first place, one can more easily relate changes in the demand for various types of health services (whether they are consumer induced or are the result of technological change) to personnel requirements. For example, the increased use of computers in medicine will in all probability affect initially the diagnostic and administrative groups (1 and 5) more than it will the others. Second, a functional grouping should make possible more meaningful cost estimates both within and outside the hospital settings. Third, functional classification can add a needed dimension of relevance to studies of wage levels, skill requirements and wage differentials.

From the point of view of recruitment of new personnel to the health field and their guidance to its multitudinous facets, still another classification criterion is important—the degree to which a given occupation involves patient contact. The nature of medical services is such that it will always contain a large element of person-to-person contact (in Weiss's typology, about 83 percent of the jobs in 1960 were so oriented) but one major consequence of the increasing division of labor and specialization of health personnel is that the proportion of occupations which do not require patient contact is increasing, mostly in the diagnostic and administrative areas. Hence, those potential workers whose preferences and aptitudes lie in a direction which is clearly away from patient contact, and who, for that reason formerly excluded the health field from their occupational choices, need a reorientation as to the nature of many interesting and rewarding health occupations where patient contact is not required.

It is not the object of the foregoing examination of classification schemes to select one or to reject others; nor is it the object to search for an "ideal" system of classification, rather it is to point to those approaches which appear to shed most light on the forces affecting the changing composition of health manpower.

Factors Affecting the Supply of Allied Health Personnel

It may be appropriate at this point to set out explicitly the general and specific factors which operated and continue to operate to further subdivide the occupational and skill spectra in health manpower, thus serving to increase the ratio of allied to total health personnel:

1. Increased demand for care—irrespective of the reasons for it, the fact is that spending for medical care is taking a larger part of consumers' disposable income over time, and in cases of very low income, government is doing the spending.

2. Increased knowledge—reference here is to advances in the basic sciences and in medicine proper, leading, for instance, to the development of new instrumentation, complex diagnostic techniques, and to new surgical procedures (e.g., open-heart surgery), all of which require additional technicians and laboratory personnel for their implementation and operation.

3. Rising costs of medical goods and services—as a consequence of recent supply and demand conditions in the market for medical goods and services, unit prices of these items have been rising generally at a greater rate than have prices of nonmedical items. This condition generates demands for increased efficiency and lower costs by large payers for medical care such as insurance companies, large corporations, large labor unions, and government agencies. To obtain a greater amount of services with existing personnel and/ or to obtain a given amount of services at lower costs entails effi-

ciency increases which in turn involve, at least partially, the substitution of less costly for more costly labor where possible. The transfer of clerical duties from registered nurses to ward clerks, mentioned in Chapter 1, is a case in point.

4. Changing locus of employment—the trend over the years is for more health services to be provided in a hospital or other institutional setting, and it is in these settings that two-thirds of all health service personnel are employed. Since allied health personnel constitute over 80 percent of total health manpower, a continuation of this trend will also serve to increase the allied health ratio. And the hospitals themselves, especially the short-term general hospitals, have been getting larger, and the larger the hospital, other things being equal, the greater the ratio of allied health to total personnel. (The larger hospital offers more facilities and a greater variety of services.)

In addition, the expansion of existing facilities such as nursing homes and the growth of newer types of facilities such as public health centers, clinics, rehabilitation facilities, neighborhood health centers, group practice facilities, and the like, all make for an increased ratio of allied health personnel.

5. Changing concepts of disease management—this factor may be summarized in the phrase "progressive patient care," and it derives from the concept of an illness continuum ranging from critical to recovered, which, in turn, necessitates a finer division of labor and of facilities. It also involves the use of separate rehabilitation facilities for ambulatory patients and in these loci, again, allied health personnel predominate.

6. Changing patterns of health care financing—in point 3 above we mentioned the concern of large payers for medical care (so-called third parties) over constantly rising costs. An additional factor is involved here—health insurance contracts, by the way they are written, encourage the use of hospitals, of auxiliary services in hospitals, and in some plans periodic checkups including EKG's,

laboratory tests, and others are encouraged, and these procedures involve allied health personnel to a large extent.

Points 1 through 6 all support the trend toward an increased utilization of allied health manpower. However, two important factors may be mentioned as having opposite effects. The first is technology. The use of an autoanalyzer, for example, means that fewer laboratory technicians may be required for certain types of tests. The use of disposables obviates or lessens the need for workers in the clean-up and sterilization phases of care. The use of computers for business data processing as well as for patient and work-force scheduling, and even in diagnosis, while still in its infancy, presages declines in demand for certain types of allied health personnel.

The second factor that may cause decreases in allied health personnel is the trend toward the contracting-out by hospitals of certain services now performed in-house, such as general maintenance, payroll processing, patient feeding, equipment leasing rather than purchase, and so on. The employees in the service firms to whom these functions are transferred are not classified as medical personnel. Moreover, the transferred occupations are often occupation rather than industry-specific.

The data which we have examined on employment growth rates, however, indicate that the tendencies toward the proliferation of new health occupations and of employment increases in existing ones far outweigh those which may exert counter effects.

CHAPTER 3

Sources of Supply

THERE ARE A NUMBER of general factors as well as special considerations that enter into a discussion of the supply of workers—first to the economy as a whole and then to a specific sector or industry. The aggregate supply of workers is affected, of course, by the whole population, its age and sex distribution, and socio-economic variables such as education laws which set or attempt to set minimum age requirements for labor-force entry and retirement rules and regulations which attempt to set maximum ones. Then there are such sociological factors as attitudes towards single or married women as workers, attitudes towards minorities, and the like. On another level there are the attitudes, customs, and practices surrounding individual occupations, such as the identification of nursing with females and surgery with males. Finally, the focus narrows to questions of availability, geographic mobility, and formal licensure or certification requirements. Actual employment occurs in a local labor market where the dominant factors are wages, hours, and working conditions.

Analyses of some of these factors as they affect allied health manpower are undertaken in the following three chapters. This chapter will deal largely with the demographic aspects of supply—that is, with the age, sex, and educational groups within the general population from which potential allied health workers may be drawn.

Some Special Features
of Allied Health Manpower Supply and Distribution

There are two characteristics of the health services and of allied health occupations in particular that must be delineated before proceeding with more detailed analyses—geographical distribution and occupational complexity.

Health workers are dispersed throughout the country in a variety of institutional settings, ranging from thousands of solo practitioners' offices to large institutions such as Bellevue Hospital Center in New York, for example, which in 1967 had 7,365 employees.[1] With the exception of the largest cities, where two independent hospitals might be next door to each other, the 7,000 hospitals are scattered throughout the country with relatively large distances between them—varying from a few miles in the populated Northeast to perhaps fifty miles in the rural Southwest.

The influence of geographic configuration alone on the distribution of health facilities is revealed by Table 3.1, which compares two states of approximately equal population.

Table 3.1

Hospital Facilities, Ohio and Texas, 1963

	Ohio	*Texas*
Population 1963	10,000,000	10,228,000
Number of hospitals (nonmilitary)	268	563
Number of communities with hospitals *	132	278
Total number of beds	81,927	70,170
Median number of beds per hospital	306	125
Median full-time personnel per hospital †	368	158
Population per bed	122	146

* Community ranges from largest city to rural location.

† Excludes residents, interns, students, and attending physicians.

Source: *Hospitals: Journal of the American Hospital Association,* Vol. 39, Part 2 (August 1, 1965), *Guide Issue.*

[1] *Hospitals: Journal of the American Hospital Association,* Vol. 41, Part 2, *Guide Issue* (August 1, 1967), p. 176.

Ohio, we may note, has fewer but larger hospitals, while Texas has more but smaller and more widely dispersed facilities. There are other industries, such as retail trade and education for example, which show greater geographic dispersion than the health services. They do not, however, require the wide range of occupations per facility that are necessary, even in small hospitals. Not only is there a large number of fairly discrete disciplines required (laboratories, X-rays, clinicians) but a wide hierarchy of skill levels within them as well. Depending on defintions, estimates of the number of separate occupations in the health field range from 37 to 102 and within the allied health worker area itself, from 21 to 53.[2]

The Narrow Locus of Training and Employment

Every employing institution draws most of its allied health workers from local people, who are trained or trainable in the required occupations. Even its student population comes mainly from the surrounding area, with the possible exception of professional nursing students. The exceptions to this local dependency are the Armed Forces hospitals, which train and assign their military workers on a national or international scale, and to a lesser extent the Catholic hospitals, which have some control over the geographical mobility of certain religious workers. However, even these institutions make heavy use of local civilian manpower.

Workers in most of the allied health occupations are relatively immobile. Although they do move for various reasons, they are not part of a continuous and free-flowing national labor market. On the whole they must be recruited from the local population and trained locally if they are to be employed in a local institution.

The special circumstances surrounding married women must be

[2] "Manpower in the 1960s," *Health Manpower Source Book,* Section 18 (Washington, Dept. of Health, Education, and Welfare, 1964); and "Health Careers Guidebook," (Washington, Dept. of Labor).

emphasized here. In cases where the husband must relocate, the wife does too, so that to some degree, female health worker mobility is a response to the incentives or pressures on her husband rather than on herself.

The large number of occupations required in a hospital means that there will often be only a few workers in any given occupation in any one institution. As a consequence, recruitment, training, and employment must be provided for dozens of occupations in hundreds of localities. This fragmentation of employment has resulted in a fragmentation of hiring standards, training programs, and staffing patterns. That most hospitals resemble each other in the general contours of staffing is largely due to the nature of the work and the state of the art. For example, mental hospital staffing patterns tend on the whole to be very similar, but to differ from the staffing patterns of general hospitals. These in turn differ from the staffing patterns of special service hospitals.

National professional organizations provide an impetus to standardization through their influence on training programs. Regulatory agencies of local, state, and federal government units also exert some influence toward standardization, but the variations within the general framework are wide and depend to a large extent on the local availability of trained and/or trainable workers.

Young Women

There is little detailed information on the sources of supply for allied health workers beyond the 1960 Census, which is now eight years out of date. Health service employment has increased rapidly since then. Between 1960 and 1965 it increased 27 percent (see Chapter 2). But all indications are that the proportions and trends described have not changed appreciably.

It is clear from an examination of Table 3.2 that the majority of health service workers are women, and a large part of them young

women. In fact, more than two-thirds of the workers in health services are women, a proportion which is the exact opposite of that in
all other industries. Several industries do use a greater proportion
of women in their work force, but only educational services and
private household services use an equal or greater number.

Table 3.2

*Workers in Health Services and
All Industries in 1960,
by Age and Sex (in percent)*

Age	Health Services		All Industries	
	F	M	F	M
Total	69.7	30.3	31.2	68.8
14 to 34 yrs.	28.1	9.4	11.5	25.1
35 to 54 yrs.	30.0	13.9	14.4	30.9
55 yrs.	11.6	7.0	5.3	12.7

Source: Adapted from *Health Manpower Source Book*, Section 17 (Washington, Dept. of Health, Education, and Welfare), Table 3, p. 7.

Using the data source for Table 3.2, we calculated that almost
10 percent of the workers in health services were women between
the ages of 20 and 24 and 12.6 percent were in the 18 to 24 age
group. This latter group then constitutes an important source of
supply because this is the age of entrance to the labor force of many
new workers.

Population projections indicate that in absolute terms, all age
and sex groups with the exception of the 35 to 44 year olds will increase by 1975.[3] But the females in the 15 to 24 year age group
will constitute not only a greater number but a relatively greater
proportion of the population in 1975 relative to that of 1960. If
these women continue to enter health service occupations in the

[3] *Statistical Abstract of the United States, 1965* (Washington, Bureau of the
Census), Table 3, p. 8.

same proportions as they do currently, their total impact will then be greater. Counter influences here are the elongation of the schooling period for this age group as well as the current trend toward a lowering of the age of marriage and possible shifts in relative wage levels.

The dominance of the feminine image over the allied health occupations stems from the fact that nurses, who were the first non-M.D. health workers, were women. Nursing and teaching were among the few professions traditionally acceptable to the parents of middle-class daughters, and for less-advantaged females, nursing provided the opportunity for stable employment, education, and social advancement.

It is generally socially acceptable in our society for men to take leadership positions and women supportive jobs. In a hospital this is largely true in that the physicians (mostly men) give the orders, and the nurses and other allied health workers (usually women) carry them out. The relatively high proportion of males in commanding positions and low proportion in subordinate positions is as follows:

	Percent Male
Physicians and surgeons (full-time staff)	90.1
Psychologists	74.1
Pharmacists	66.8
Chemists	57.1
Biological scientists	47.1
Therapists and healers	38.0
Technicians, medical and dental	31.4
Attendants	27.9

Most allied health jobs are characterized by low wages and lack of advancement. Both of these conditions are associated with a high rate of female participation, especially young females without families to support. The shortage of allied health workers is seen as an advantage to them because "you can always get a job if you want one." Conversely, for a certain segment of this group the lack of advancement possibilities is not seen as a serious disadvantage, because most of the young women expect to be working only until they marry and have children.

The Effect of Female Concentration

The high concentration of women in health services has several effects on allied health manpower. For one thing, as has already been implied, men are reluctant to enter fields dominated by women. More important, the high concentration of young women is associated with a high dropout rate as the young women marry and "retire" from the labor force to raise families. For example, a survey of dental hygienists by the American Council on Education showed that 46 percent of the respondents were not employed, the majority of these, 79.5 percent, giving "family obligations" as the reason.[4] In another case, the American Dietetics Association found, in a survey of its membership, that among the respondents of child-rearing ages, between 44 and 51 percent were not working in dietetics, and that of this group less than half had worked for more than five years in dietetics.[5] (It should be pointed out that 83 percent of those not working were planning to return to work within ten years.)

Information is not readily available for other occupations in such detail. One tabulation in the 1960 Census showed that in several medical occupations there were relatively high proportions in what was termed the "labor reserve," defined as those between the ages 14 and 54 who last worked in a given occupation between 1950 and 1960. Thus, about 37 percent of medical and dental technicians, 28 percent of therapists, and 23 percent of practical nurses

[4] Robert G. Kessel and M. Holinquist, "Survey of Dentistry: Report on Dental Hygienists," *American Dental Hygienist Association*, 35–37 (January 1961), 13.

[5] "A Look at Ourselves," *Journal of the American Dietetic Association*, 41 (December 1962), 537–41.

and midwives were listed as being in the labor reserve category. The ratios of ex-workers in these allied health fields exceeded those for accountants, secondary school teachers, and social workers.[6]

Not only is there a large pool of former health employees but almost all of the hospitals report high turnover rates among existing personnel. It is, of course, to be expected that turnover rates will be higher in industries and occupations where the labor supply is taut than in situations where unemployment rates are high. Undoubtedly this is an additional factor in the allied health field apart from the age–sex ratio. High turnover rates add significantly to operating costs. They also contribute to low morale (as well as being in part caused by it). And ultimately, high turnover rates have an adverse effect on patient care. A more detailed examination of data on hospital turnover rates is reserved for Chapter 6.

Older Women

Women who leave the labor force to raise families frequently return to work after their children begin to grow up. Many women who trained for health services in the 1940s and 1950s are now available for reemployment. The largest increase in labor force participation rate for the past two decades has in fact occurred among women in the 45 to 54 age group. The cycle therefore for a large part of the female population is: training and work during the teens and early twenties, retirement from the labor force when children arrive and until the children begin to grow up or are "grown," and then reentry into the labor force at middle age, presumably into the same occupation trained for and/or worked in during the first time period.[7]

Only recently are health officials becoming aware of and willing

[6] "United States Summary," *U.S. Census of Population, 1960,* "Detailed Characteristics," Table 205, and "Occupational Characteristics," Table 20.

[7] *Manpower Report of the President, 1966,* p. 154.

to use these women. Unfortunately the intervening period has seen tremendous changes in the provision of health services, and many of the women find their skills not only blunted but obsolete. Retraining programs, such as those under the auspices of the Manpower Development and Training Act and the American Hospital Association are already in operation. But frequently these are only temporary or ad hoc affairs, instituted to deal with particularly severe shortages and are terminated when the shortage is abated or the monetary grant is exhausted. It should be recognized that entry, dropout, and reentry is a predictable, on-going pattern for a large part of the female labor force, and that reentrants to the labor force are not a source to be drawn on in emergency only but are constantly available resources to be utilized on a continuous basis. A study by the National League for Nursing in 1962 showed for instance, that 21 percent of the practical nursing students were over 34 years old and that 10 percent of the students were widowed, divorced, or separated.[8]

Retraining programs, rather than being one-time efforts, could be permanently institutionalized and would provide for an important source of workers. Montague Brown of the New Jersey Hospital Research–Educational Trust, emphasized the importance of retraining programs. He estimated that the New Jersey nursing schools graduate only about 1,000 nurses a year, of whom about half leave within a few years. Recent nurse-refresher programs turned out 600 nurses in a year, most of whom are expected to remain in nursing for fairly long periods. If such programs were institutionalized they would become recognized by the potential returnees as a means of reentering their occupations, and one that would provide an opportunity to relearn jobs before having to perform them. The mere existence of such an opportunity is often sufficient to persuade people to utilize it.

[8] Barbara Tate, "Nursing Students: Who Are They?" (New York, National League for Nursing, 1962).

Most of the refresher or retraining programs instituted so far have been for professional nurses rather than for other allied health personnel. Hopefully these programs will be broadened in the future.

Educational Prerequisites

Most medical and allied health occupations require a period of specialized training, either before employment or immediately upon first becoming employed. As in most industries, the least desirable jobs go to those with the least training. Almost all jobs require some training and some minimum general education prior to specific occupational training.

For example, in most states one cannot begin training as a nurse without a high-school diploma, and one cannot normally begin training as a physician without a baccalaureate degree. So these are the educational jumping-off points for health service work in these two occupations.

In the lowest level jobs—aides, attendants, orderlies—there are no educational requirements. There are also no training requirements. Licensed practical nurses are required by law in twenty-seven states to have completed the tenth grade, and in ten states to have completed high school. Five states require ninth-grade and eight require eighth-grade completion. Most of the therapy and technical occupations require a minimum of high-school graduation.

With few exceptions the prerequisite general education and the point of entry into allied health training is high-school graduation. It is both the minimum requirement and the maximum requirement; without a high-school diploma it is difficult to advance beyond the level of an unskilled worker. The only skilled occupation which does not require high-school graduation is practical nursing. For the remainder of the allied health occupations the source of supply is largely the high-school graduate, either at the time of graduation or before any further education or training can be undertaken.

The Training System

Another factor limiting the supply of allied health workers is the formal training system itself. It is perhaps overcomplimentary to call it a system. More accurately it could be described as a loosely connected set of independent programs, each under the aegis of its professional society, all subject to the general approval of the joint interprofessional committees, of which the American Medical and American Dental Associations are the most prominent members, and subject to the influence of the hospital or school which sponsors the program. In addition there are a variety of programs and schools not approved by these committees, and a variety of training efforts which could not be called programs in any strict sense (see Chapter 4).

The approved programs however usually are those which get publicity and funds, public and private, and the graduates of these are acceptable employees in most hospitals. Although one can hold a job without having taken an approved program, one would have difficulty building a career without it. Therefore the source of supply of "lifetime" workers is largely limited to the people willing and able to take approved training.

There are then three special characteristics of allied health manpower. First, the vast majority of workers are young women; second, the point of entrance is high-school graduation; third, the route of entry is through an approved training program. Each of these limits the supply of potential workers. The present concern for increasing the number of workers requires that attention be paid to increasing the flow from each of these sources and on developing new programs of the informal or on-the-job training variety.

Increasing the Supply

The number of young women who go into health services must be measured against the number who enter other occupations.

One way to arrive at the job alternatives available to young women is to examine the average educational attainment of workers in different occupations. An analysis of the data in the Occupational Characteristics volume of the 1960 Census reveals, for example, that women in the 20 to 24 year age group who are hospital attendants had a median educational attainment of 10.2 years. These young women could conceivably have been checkers and inspectors —occupations in which the educational levels were equal—or counter and fountain workers or assemblers, where the median level was only one month more (10.3 years). Practical nurses attained an educational level of 11.1. These women could perhaps have also been sales ladies and sales clerks where the level was 11.4 or 4 months higher, and most certainly they could have entered those occupations which were lower in the educational scale. Attendants in physicians' and dentists' offices had a 12.5 educational level, equal to that recorded for receptionists, typists, and bookkeepers. It is interesting to note that medical and dental technicians attained a median education level of 13.2, exactly the same as that for professional nurses and dieticians. Presumably some fluidity among these occupations is possible. Elementary-school teachers, with whom professional nurses are often compared, had a 16.4 level compared with the 13.2 for the RN's. Most striking are the clusters at 12.5 and 13.2 years of median education. Professional nursing, it would appear, is the biggest competitor for the dietician and technician.

Efforts have been made from time to time, to attract males into the health services industry. Administrators, recognizing the volatility of a largely feminine labor supply, hoped that male workers would be more likely to remain in the industry and show greater commitment to their careers. An effort after World War II to convert medical corpsmen into practical nurses did not succeed and most efforts to attract males into the nursing occupations since then have also been failures. Nursing is "women's work" and appears likely to remain so for a long time.

An increasing number of technician and therapist jobs, however, has added to the number of male workers, even though the increase in female workers has far overshadowed them. A large increase in male workers would require not only recruitment efforts but basic changes in the employment structure. Men would be attracted to a stable lifelong career commitment only with higher salaries, advancement opportunities, and independent job responsibilities.

High-school graduation as a prerequisite for employment and training poses many problems. The most common census occupational category for female high-school graduates is "clerical and kindred." Although wages are not particularly high in these occupations, the skills can be learned fairly quickly, training is frequently available as part of the high-school curriculum, the work is clean, and the hours are regular. Lower-level health occupations on the whole do not offer comparable advantages, given the ease of entering clerical work.

High-school dropouts are utilized in unskilled health service jobs but are prevented from rising to better jobs by their lack of the prerequisite diploma or certificate. Incorporating into these jobs, some academic training, leading at least to a high-school equivalency diploma would be of great assistance to many of these employees. Practical nursing is one of the few allied health occupations requiring fairly extensive training (approximately one year) that does not require high-school graduation as a prerequisite to training. In fact, many practical nursing courses are given within high school as part of the vocational education programs, or in vocational and technical institutions for high-school graduates and nongraduates alike.

A person who has not graduated from high school is not necessarily unable to benefit from extensive job training or unable to undertake training as a skilled worker or technician. Motivation is an important consideration, as is experience in other fields. Furthermore it must be noted that the older generation of women now available for training and employment does not have as much formal schooling on the whole as has the younger generation. A sliding educational requirement such as that now in use in several states for practical nursing may be an approach to this problem. In Arizona, for example, the law states that an applicant for practical nursing training must have completed ten grades in school if she is under 25 years old, but need only have completed eight grades if she is over 25. Such sliding requirements in other occupations and at other educational levels would be generally useful in widening the source of supply of future workers.

Training programs which are sponsored by the various professional associations are, as we have pointed out, an important source of new health workers. However, the prerequisite educational requirements tend to be relatively high. It is therefore very important, if we are to augment the supply of allied health workers, to explore the possibilities of lowering the educational requirements for many types of workers or to develop new training programs for interested groups or for occupations which are emerging as a result of new technologies. We must also experiment with varieties of sponsorship: hospitals, ambulatory centers, government—as in the military, in the Manpower Training and Development Act (MDTA) and in the Office of Economic Opportunity (OEO)—junior colleges, and secondary schools and institutions.

The so-called "New Careers" program sponsored by a consortium of federal agencies—Department of Labor, Department of Health, Education and Welfare, Office of Economic Opportunity, Department of Housing and Urban Development—aims at the creation of such entry level jobs with built-in mobility features, many of which are in the health occupations.

Summary

Positions in the allied health field are mainly filled by females, most of whom first enter this area when young. This has important effects on the structure of employment, the most important of which for present discussion is that young females retire from the labor force to raise families. This causes a high labor force dropout rate in the industry. Given the present pattern of female participation in work —training, entry, dropout, and reentry—it becomes obvious that an important source of manpower is the reentry pool. Developing retraining programs to accommodate older women would increase the flow from this increasingly important source of supply.

The concentration on high-school graduation as the entry point into eventual health employment results from a complex of factors which will be examined in more detail in the next chapter. There are requirements for education which are minimally necessary for job performance, there are qualifications preferred by employers, and there are requirements which are formally demanded by the institutions involved. The professional societies, among others, are concerned with keeping quality and wages high. For some of the low-skilled occupations, where the supply is most taut, high-school graduation is the minimum prerequisite. For some of the low-skilled occupations, where potential supply is greater, high-school graduation would appear to be an unnecessarily high requirement.

Technological and organizational changes are however, speeding up the division of labor in many instances generating new jobs on all skill levels and requiring a wide variety of educational prerequisites.

Since the labor market for allied health workers is quite unstructured (see Chapter 5) the institutionally demanded qualifications are often lowered to the preferred or even the minimally necessary level. Given the high turnover rates and the rapid expansion of the health fields, hospital administrators have found it necessary to utilize their work force under conditions of limited education, limited training, limited skill transferability, and tight supervision. This provides workers for specific jobs in specific hospitals, but not meaningful lifetime careers which would be attractive to well-trained men beginning their working lives.

CHAPTER 4

Education and Training

EVERY INDUSTRY needs workers trained in the job skills peculiar to that industry. Most job-oriented skills are learned in high schools and colleges or through training received on the job. Formal training programs or apprenticeships sponsored by companies, industries, or craft union organizations are on the whole a relatively minor part of the American educational scene. Allied health training is characterized by extensive dependence on this latter type of training. This is partly due to the specialized type of knowledge needed in health care, and partly due to historical development.

Historical Development

As outlined in Chapter 2, the trained work force of a hospital fifty years ago was composed of doctors and nurses. The tasks that are now performed by trained allied health workers were then either not performed at all or performed as part of the regular duties of the doctors and nurses. When other workers were needed, "a strong back and a weak mind" would usually suffice. Training of allied health personnel is a more recent development than the training of doctors and nurses, and to some extent was patterned after and influenced by the methods employed in the education of these personnel.

Originally both doctors and nurses learned their jobs by watching and imitating experienced practitioners and practicing under a watchful eye. Formal training even for these professions is relatively recent. The first Nightingale schools for nurses in the United States were not founded until 1873.[1] Around the turn of the century many doctors were still being trained by the preceptor or apprenticeship method.[2] But the systems of formal education under which now all doctors and professional nurses are trained were fairly well established by the end of World War I. The two forms of schooling associated with the two occupations represent the alternative models for allied health training.

Partly under the influence of the Flexner Report of 1910, the training of medical students was seen as the province of a university, largely theoretical and abstract with the practical technique picked up along the way. Students were expected to pay the university for their education. On the other hand, nursing schools from the beginning were associated with hospitals, if not owned outright by them. The training was practical and experiential with the theory picked up along the way, and students were paid a stipend and perquisites from the beginning of their study.

Despite the differing approaches, the two types of schooling had in common a concern with theory, the practical application of theory, and the development of particular job skills. Both required that a large part of the student's time be spent in ward practice.

As the need for more and different types of workers grew, the history of their training followed that of doctors and nurses. The first workers were trained on the job; only later did formal schooling begin.

It would be too lengthy here to detail the origins of the various allied health workers. Most originated as assistants to doctors or

[1] Isabel Maitland Stewart, *The Education of Nurses* (New York, Macmillan, 1943).

[2] Lowell T. Coggeshall, "Planning for Medical Progress through Education," (Evanston, Ill., American Association of Medical Assistants, April 1965).

other health professionals and eventually rose to the technical or subprofessional level;[3] some developed from traditional occupations or trades to become bona fide professionals themselves;[4] still others started as workers in other industries and later found a place in health work.[5]

The early developments in allied health training were mainly restricted to training on the job or in a job related setting, rather than in schools. Very common was a short "probationary" period on the job. The worker was either unpaid or very poorly paid, and he received minimal instructions and maximal practice until he was considered "trained." The cost to the hospital was relatively low, consisting mainly of a few hours of "instructor's" time, and the benefits in terms of work performed by the student were great. (Such apprenticeship arrangements were quite common in many industries in the eighteenth and nineteenth centuries.)

Much of the work that is now performed by allied health personnel was performed by volunteers for charitable or ideological purposes. For example, the first pathologist in New York City was so poorly esteemed by his colleagues that he had to rent his own laboratory space at Presbyterian Hospital. But students and others who believed in this new form of medicine voluntarily staffed the laboratory in order to sit at the foot of the great man and help him accomplish his mission. They received a free education and he received free laboratory assistants.

However as an occupation becomes routinized and accepted, volunteers cannot be relied on forever. A common way to obtain trained manpower is to let someone else do the training. For many

[3] For example, the pamphlet *History of the American Association of Medical Assistants* (Chicago, American Association of Medical Assistants, n.d.).

[4] For example, M. E. Cox, *Optometry, the Profession: Its Antecedents, Birth, and Development* (Philadelphia, Chilton, 1957).

[5] For example, many of the earliest nuclear technicians were trained by the government during World War II. As radio-isotopes were developed for medical purposes, this occupation became part of the health manpower scene.

years physicians and dentists in private practice have used office assistants who received their clerical training either in high school or in nonhealth industries. Many of the newer workers in the health field such as computer analysts and nuclear medicine technologists are recruited from other industries.

There were many factors influencing the emergence of formal training among allied health workers. As the health services industry expanded a greater proportion of its manpower was in the nonprofessional and allied health categories. It was no longer a case of skill acquisition for one or two people but for up to three-quarter's of the hospital staff (see Chapter 1). The expansion of medical knowledge combined with the increased demand for services made such specialization necessary.

As the work force grew, the desire for economic and social status also grew and the workers in the various occupations began forming into professional organizations. The main push toward organization followed World War I, as follows:

1847	American Medical Association
1896	American Nurses Association
	American Dental Association
1912	American Podiatry Association
1917	American Dietetics Association
1918	American Optometric Association
1920	American Society of Radiologic Technologists
1925	American Dental Assistant Association
1925	American Speech and Hearing Association
1925	American Psychological Association
1928	American Association of Medical Record Librarians
1928	American Society of Medical Technologists
	American Occupational Therapy Association
	Medical Orthotics and Prosthetics Association
	National Association of Social Workers
	American Dental Hygiene Association
1956	American Association of Medical Assistants

Changing technology required workers better trained than the unskilled assistants, and the workers themselves desired better training which would lead to a more important place for the occupation in the medical fields.

Many of the physicians and other higher level professionals also found that well-trained assistants were worth the investment, and took it upon themselves to sponsor training programs for the fledgling occupations. The dental profession was especially quick to sponsor training programs for dental personnel.

A natural outgrowth of the unpaid apprenticeship method was the formalization of hospital-based training similar to the system in use for nurses' training. The majority of programs cost the student nothing and most institutions pay a modest stipend during the training period. The faculty is usually recruited from the staff of the hospitals, either the physicians in charge of the department or the already trained allied health workers. In university or teaching hospitals, the programs are usually under the direction of the clinical professor in the specialty.

The desire for status as well as for higher incomes generated the drive for formal academic degrees and accredited programs which would certify the worker as a well-trained "professional."

The independent emergence of college education as a goal for the majority of youth, and later the use of junior colleges as training institutions, gave impetus to the change toward formal education for workers.

Most of the allied health occupations require some knowledge of the biological or chemical sciences; others require a knowledge of psychology and other social sciences. Instruction in these subjects, including some experience in laboratory techniques, is largely the province of the higher educational institutions rather than of the industries requiring the skills. Those occupations which chose this route followed the model of physicians' training.

These two types of programs—the hospital based and the university based—are the most prevalent. However, there are a multitude of smaller-scale training efforts which are combinations of the two or slight variants of them. Most include either the extension of formal education into new occupations or the diversification of the types of institutions giving the training. Among the former are programs for nurse's aides and surgical technicians; among the latter are programs under MDTA and the vocational school system. Despite the growth of formal training there are still many jobs, and many presently evolving occupations, in which the workers are trained on the job, either explicitly or implicitly.

Present Structure

The present structure of allied health training includes all the various patterns. It might be useful for analytical purposes to make a distinction between education and training. Education is directed toward acquiring general knowledge applicable to a wide variety of situations and frequently is only indirectly related to a vocational objective. Training is taken to acquire the specific skills needed in a specific job or occupation, whether these skills be physical or mental. Education and training are not, however, entirely separate. Some education provides a background of knowledge which is relevant to the occupation. A proper mastery of technique during training requires some understanding of the principles involved.

The relative proportions of education and training deemed necessary for a job influences the type of training given and the institutional setting in which it is given. Practical training, or clinical training as it is called in this industry, must be given either on the job or in a job-like setting, as it is necessary for the student to familiarize himself with the actual tools, machines, and procedures used in his work. Theoretical (didactic) training does not usually require extensive practical equipment; its tools (apart from teachers) are textbooks, blackboards, and chalk. Such classroom training is not tied to the clinical setting and can be given in a variety of settings and educational institutions.

At the present time there are no comprehensive data on the extent of allied health training in the United states. The Division of Vocational and Technical Education of Health, Education, and Welfare in its first survey (1966) of nonprofessional programs in health occupations located 1,259 nonprofit institutions that have at least one active program for a total of 1,685 programs in 42 occupations. Their listing excludes all occupations requiring bachelors' or higher degrees, excludes all private and commercial schools, and excludes all on-the-job or in-service training programs.

Since there are no comprehensive statistics on trainees or programs in these excluded categories, it is not feasible to attempt to determine the relative importance of each type of training. However, the list of schools (Table 4.1) in those health occupations for which information is available, gives some indication of the importance of each type of institution. The major institutions are hospital schools and higher educational institutions. Their importance is even greater when consideration is given to on-the-job training programs in hospitals and to science courses in colleges which often lead to health jobs, but which are not included in this tabulation.

This list is far from complete. For one thing, some of the programs included exist only on paper; for another, many programs which are not accredited by professional societies are not included. Third, a variety of training institutions such as MDTA, private trade schools, vocational schools, and military are not listed.

Hospitals are probably the most important institutions in health service training. Since hospitals are the major institutions requiring allied health manpower, on-the-job training became a device for obtaining trained workers, or at least was looked upon as such by the hospital. The extent to which students who have been trained in a given hospital tend to remain as workers in that hospital is not known with any precision. Evidence seems to indicate that a large portion of the workers do so. For example, a program designed to

Table 4.1

*Educational Programs in Selected Health Occupations,
by Category of Personnel and Type of Institution,* 1965*

Category of Personnel	Total	Univ. with Med. Sch.	Other Univ. †	4-Yr. Coll.	Jr. Coll.	Tech. or Voc. Sch.	Second-ary Sch.	Hosp. or Lab.	Independ. Sch.
Med. record librarian	29	11	3	8				7	
Med. technol.	692	63	127	349	19			133	1
Occupational therapist	32	21	6	5					
Physical therapist	42	37	2					3	
Speech therapist	152	43	53	56					
Dental hygienist	55	29	7	3	15				1
Radiologic technol.	693	44	17	29	31			579	
Social worker	60	44	15	1					
Nurse	1,170	63	64	102	123			781	37
Cytotechnol.	75	26						48	1
Inhalation therapist	25	1			4			20	
Dental asst.	94	7	3	3	47	30		2	2
Dental lab. technician	11	2	1		3	5			
Lab. technician, asst.	147	2			10	16		118	1
Practical nurse	1,002	1	7	9	133	549	60	239	11
Med. asst.	43		1	1	28	13			
Med. record technician	14				2			12	
Surgical technician	12				1	5		6	
Dietician's asst.	4				2	1		1	

* Includes institutions in fifty states, District of Columbia, and Puerto Rico.

† Either offering doctoral or master's degree and having a program in liberal arts with one or more professional schools.

Source: Compiled from data in "Health Resource Statistics: Health Manpower, 1965," *Public Health Service Publication No. 1509* (Washington, 1966), 182 pp. and unpublished sources.

upgrade licensed practical nurses to the level of registered nurses at the Hospital for Joint Diseases in New York City graduated 23 students in its first class in 1966. Nineteen of these remained at that hospital although they were under no formal obligation to do so. The New York Hospital estimates that of an average class of 18 in its X-ray technology school, 8 to 12 remain at the hospital. How long they remain is an open question.

Since hospitals are working institutions, the training tends to be practical or clinical with the emphasis on experience. This is a cost advantage for the hospital, since a good deal of routine work is done by unpaid or poorly paid students. Among the voluntary general hospitals in New York City belonging to the United Hospital Fund, the average number of full-time graduate and practical nurses per 100 beds for hospitals with 200 to 299 beds was 36.6; for hospitals in this category with schools of nursing, the average was only 32.3. For 300 to 400-bed hospitals, the average number of full-time personnel in X-ray and X-ray therapy was 5.8; for those with schools of X-ray technology attached, the average was only 4.1.[6] The gap in full-time staffing is thus partly filled by student manpower.

Comprehensive cost–benefit analyses of hospital schools have not been undertaken. Most hospital schools are either free to the student or cost, at most, a few hundred dollars, and many pay stipends to the trainee. Some of the analyses, however, which have been made of nursing schools show that the training costs to the hospitals are greater than the benefits derived from the utilization of low-cost student manpower.[7]

In the meantime hospitals, under intense pressure to keep their costs low, have sometimes resisted moving the training programs out of their institutions because they fear that the costs of student

[6] United Hospital Fund of New York, *Analysis of Hospital Personnel,* Supplement III: *Financial and Statistical Analysis,* 1964.

[7] Herbert Klarman, *Hospital Care in New York City* (New York, Columbia University Press, 1963).

manpower are not as great as would be the costs of fully trained workers. Moreover, they feel that they may not obtain all of the workers they need in the open market.

Another type of hospital-based program is on-the-job training for new employees. Given the high labor force dropout rates and the expanding need for workers, employers cannot always afford to wait for the accredited training programs to turn out the workers needed, if, indeed, there are any accredited programs available. The solution is frequently to use well-trained workers in the same field or in a more highly trained field to teach the new worker his job. Thus a laboratory assistant may learn her task from another laboratory assistant or from a medical technician under whom she works.

The second large category of training institutions is composed of colleges and universities. Several of the allied health occupations are restricted to the graduates of formal college programs. Among them are dental hygiene, occupational and physical therapy, psychology, and pharmacy. Pharmacy is taught in separate schools; the others are usually departments within colleges or universities. In most states one cannot become a member of these occupational groups without having completed a legally or professionally prescribed academic training curriculum.

Junior or community colleges, in particular those supported by public funds, consider it part of their mandate to educate and train workers for essential jobs in their communities. The American Association of Junior Colleges reports programs in 40 health occupations, the most prevalent of which are the 136 nursing programs, 93 dental assisting programs, and 51 dental hygiene programs. In addition, many people trained in the sciences, particularly biology and chemistry, in the colleges and junior colleges are employable in the laboratories and clinics without additional formalized health training.

Vocational high schools and public vocational and technical institutes also perform much of the allied health training, usually in programs requiring one year or less in such occupations as practical nurse, dental assistant, medical laboratory assistant, X-ray technician, and physical and occupational therapy assistant. The 1,685 programs in 42 occupations mentioned earlier are all partially funded by the U.S. Office of Vocational and Technical Education.

In the past three years many new training programs have arisen under the auspices of MDTA for unemployed or underemployed workers. These are mainly institutional or school training programs, but include some on-the-job training programs as well. About 13,000 positions have been approved for on-the-job training from February, 1963, through June, 1966. The following figures, from *Employment Service Review* (November, 1966) show trainees enrolled in MDTA institutional courses in health occupations, September, 1962 through June, 1966.

Occupation	Enrollment
Total	40,714
Dental assistant	786
Dental hygienist	21
Dental laboratory technician	161
Electrocardiograph technician	9
Electroencephalograph technician	8
First aid attendant	20
Home health aide	453
Child care attendant	104
Cottage parent	34
Inhalation therapist	78
Medical assistant	59
Medical laboratory assistant	507
Medical record technician	76
Nurse's aide/Orderly	18,101
Nurse, practical licensed	15,614
Nurse, professional (refresher)	1,847
Occupational therapy aide	131
Optometrist	1
Orthoptist	78
Physical therapist	159

Occupation	Enrollment
Physical therapy attendant	17
Psychiatric aide	1,570
Radiation monitor	40
Radiologic technologist	116
Surgical technician	638
Hospital maid	86

The majority of the trainees are in courses lasting less than twenty-five weeks with a cost per enrollee of approximately $1,500 (see also Chapter 7).

There are also many commercial or private trade schools. These schools received great impetus from the G.I. Bill after World War II. Although they are more likely to specialize in mechanical skills and business trades, they also turn out some allied health workers, most commonly, laboratory technicians and medical and dental assistants. There is no comprehensive information available on the number of graduates yearly, nor is there a trade association which includes all of the proprietary schools. W. A. Goodard of the National Association of Trade and Technical Schools, with 108 members, estimates conservatively that there are at least 250 schools that are doing some auxiliary health training, the majority concentrating on the training of medical assistants. The length and cost of training varies from school to school. For example although medical assistant courses are usually about 1,200 class hours, one national chain of private schools gives a course of only 400 hours duration. Tuition costs range from $500 to $1,800 depending on the school and the duration of the course.

Many health educators and administrators object to the presence of profit-making schools in the health services industry. However, these schools do provide training for occupations in which nonprofit programs are lacking. Only in the past three or four years have any publicly sponsored or nonprofit programs come into being for medical office assistants or medical laboratory technicians, and even now these are few in number. The approved training institutions frequently lag behind the industry in terms of types of courses offered, whereas the private schools make every effort to stay ahead and to respond quickly to changes in demand.

Another source of training is the military. Each service trains the majority of its own lower-level and intermediate-level personnel, although training requirements are usually waived for those previously trained in civilian life. The doctors, dentists, and nurses enter upon military duty already trained. However, training in some specialities may be acquired in the service.

Evaluation of Allied Health Training

Given the lack of precise information on even the number of schools, it is impossible to find more than impressionistic data on several important aspects of training. Among these are the extent to which the schools are or are not filled to capacity, the variability in the length of courses, the variable coverage of the subject matter, the influence of professionally approved educational programs, and the qualifications of the staff.

The capacity of the various training programs, both civilian and military and the extent to which they are utilized to capacity is difficult to determine. The few figures given below would indicate that the number of students could be increased with the existing facilities, though the figures are not fully reliable. The New York State Committee on Medical Education found in 1962 that physical therapy schools in the nation were running at 77 percent of capacity and those in New York State at 52 percent of capacity. The state's occupational therapy schools were also operating at about 50 percent of capacity. It is probable that these ratios have improved since then.[8] Still, these figures contrast with the nation's graduate schools

---

[8] N.Y. State Dept. of Education, *Education for the Health Professions,* a report to the governor and the Board of Regents from the N.Y. State Committee on Medical Education (Albany, 1963).

of social work which were at 98 percent of capacity.[9] A study in Georgia in the same year found that state schools of medical technology had room for an additional 20 percent, those of X-ray technology 12 percent, and schools of practical nursing almost 50 percent.[10]

The American Society of Radiologic Technologists estimates that the majority of its schools are operating close to capacity. The American Association of Junior Colleges finds that the dental hygiene courses at its member schools are filled without difficulty while active recruitment is necessary for the other health occupations offerings. The reasons for underutilization of existing programs vary from geographic inaccessibility to financial constraints, and from lack of desirable career opportunities to the presence of better opportunities through a different, equally accessible training program. Also important is simply lack of knowledge of a program's availability.

There is great variability in the length of the training programs. For example, within the institutional courses under MDTA, nurse's aide and orderly programs range in duration from three to forty-one weeks, with concentrations at four to six weeks. This diversity is due in part to the educational needs of the workers (e.g., remedial work) as well as to the employment needs of the hospitals. However, the length of courses in programs specifically oriented toward increasing the employability of the trainees also varies greatly.

There are no exact measures of how much education is "needed" to do various jobs. Professional societies, which are concerned with raising the quality of the worker, as well as with limiting supply, attempt continually to raise the formal education requirements, as an

[9] Dept. of Health, Education, and Welfare, "Closing the Gap in Social Work Manpower," *Report of the Departmental Task Force on Social Work Education and Manpower* (Washington, November 1963).

[10] Cameron Fincher, *Nursing and Paramedical Personnel in Georgia* (Atlanta, Georgia State College, 1962).

examination of the changing certification procedures for most professional societies will reveal. Schools and colleges tend to feel that their students need more general education rather than more vocational training. Hospitals and professional medical workers, frequently more concerned with quantity than quality, tend to set the formal requirements lower, and to prefer practical training to theoretical knowledge.

For example, of the accredited dental assistant programs in 1965, the length of the programs in weeks was distributed as shown in Table 4.2.

Table 4.2

Duration of Training in Dental Assistant Programs

	Technical Institutes and Hospitals		Universities and Colleges	
	Number	*Percent*	*Number*	*Percent*
36 weeks or less	9	36	13	30
37 to 52 weeks	15	60	7	16
53 to 71 weeks	0	0	4	9
72 weeks or more	1	4	20	45
	25	100	44	100

Source: *Dental Students' Register, 1965–66* (Chicago, American Dental Association, 1966).

The greater length of the university and college programs is mainly due to the larger amount of prescribed general education. Variation can also depend on the amount of clinical practice required. For example, the official X-ray technology course given in hospitals takes two years, while the Army, which includes only didactic training, turns out X-ray technicians in twenty weeks.

The presence of a professionally approved training system does not guarantee that all workers will in practice meet these qualifications. In 1962, the New York State Department of Labor found that professional society accreditation, which usually represents the greatest amount of education, was required for only a minority of workers. "Such accreditation was specified as a minimum job requirement for 18 percent of medical records librarians, 14 percent of X-ray technicians, 4 percent of medical laboratory technologists, and 7 percent of occupational therapists. In addition there were a number of employers who expressed a preference for workers with accreditation but did not require it." [11]

State licenses were required of dental hygienists and physical therapists, all of whom met the professional society requirements. Since that time licenses have become mandatory for X-ray technicians in the state and for medical laboratory technicians in New York City; licenses required for the latter, however, are currently far below the license requirements of the American Society of Medical Technologists.

A major problem raised by the increase in training programs is the need for the rapid expansion of teaching manpower. There is very little information available on the qualifications possessed by teachers of health subjects. The "Essentials of an Accredited Curriculum" for training programs for each of the occupations accredited by the AMA include faculty requirements. The director of the program must be either an experienced and qualified practitioner of the occupation or a physician certified in the specialty being taught, and there must be at least one additional qualified practitioner. The only other formal requirement is that the teaching staff should be "competent." The Office of Vocational Education reports that nearly all of the teachers for health occupations under its jurisdiction are holders of academic degrees, a large number being nurses with baccalaureate degrees. Each state sets its own qualifications for permanent teachers although two-week preservice courses and inservice training programs are available for all beginning teachers.

---

[11] N.Y. State Dept. of Labor, *Technical Manpower in New York State; Special Bulletin 239,* Vol. II (December 1964).

The teachers of the various allied health specialties in college and junior colleges are expected to possess academic degrees for appointment. However, the rapid expansion of programs and the shortage of qualified practitioners holding academic degrees has led to the utilization of nondegree holders for many courses.

Table 4.3

New York State College
Teachers of Selected Technologies

Technology	Percent with Bachelor's Degree or Higher	
	General	Science or Technology
Dental lab. technology	24.1	10.3
Dental hygiene	61.1	46.7
X-ray technology	76.1	48.9
Medical lab. technology	86.1	81.0

A New York State Department of Labor survey, *Technical Manpower in New York State,* showed the shortage of degree holders among college and junior college teachers in 1962 (Table 4.3).

Rising Importance of Higher Education

The major development in allied health training over the past twenty years has been the increasing importance of colleges and junior colleges as training institutions. As was pointed out at the beginning of this chapter, physician education for the past fifty years in this country has been allied to universities with a prime emphasis on theoretical aspects.

The occupations listed in Table 4.1 that were trained exclusively in colleges and universities have for the most part been trained in an academic setting ever since their inception as formal programs. Although nurses training began as practical, clinical experience, it too has moved toward formal education. The numbers are still small, but as can be seen from Table 4.4 the growth of baccalaureate and associate degree nursing programs in the colleges and junior colleges has been growing over the past twenty years.

Table 4.4

Graduates of Nursing Programs

	Number of Graduates, 1964–65	Percent Increase since 1960–61
Diploma	26,795	6
Associate Degree	2,510	174
Baccalaureate	5,381	33

Source: *Facts About Nursing, 1966,* Table 6, p. 85.

As medical services have become more technologically advanced the untrained aide or casually trained assistant has had to give way to the well-trained technician. Some of the pressure comes from the workers themselves. Since the amount of education deemed necessary helps determine the prestige of any occupation there is pressure from within to raise the requirements. College education has more prestige than industrial training, and acquiring an education frequently takes precedence over learning a useful vocation. One of the reasons for the increasing popularity of the junior or community college has been its combination of general education and vocational training for those youth unable, for various reasons, to attend four-year colleges. The institution of collegiate training takes the burden of training costs from the hospitals, which are under pressure to keep their expenses down. The vocational schools, the technical institutes, and the junior colleges consider it a part of their mandate to educate and train workers needed in the local area, and indeed, these schools receive much of their funds for this express purpose. Total government expenditures for vocational education in health occupations for 1965 were $20 million, of which $14 million were from state and local funds. Although the published figures do not break down expenditures by type of institution, the enrollment by type of program gives a clue to the predominance of junior colleges and other post-secondary programs in health occupations compared to other vocational programs.[12] Junior and community colleges entered the health training picture within the past ten years, but progress has been rapid, as the figures cited earlier indicate.

Students' Choices of Training Career

So far this examination of allied health training has focused on the training structure. But there is one important influence on the dynamics of the structure which is frequently overlooked—the students.

Individuals' reasons for undertaking education and training in a particular field vary. Some have a long time-perspective—they embark on training because they want to go into the field for which the training prepares them. They may have worked in the field already and wish now to raise their occupational level; they may be recent high-school graduates with no work experience but with clear career goals. But their focus is on the field as a goal, and the training as a means. Some are focused on a different goal—getting an education—and the work for which it is preparing them, if any, is secondary to obtaining the degree. Upon graduation, they seek a job that fits their qualifications. They are not likely to have taken particularly specialized courses and will only be available for jobs which require general education. Especially among women, who form such a large part of the allied health work force, a B.A. or an A.A. is not so much a professional as a social and personal prerequisite. The number of college graduates attending secretarial

[12] U.S. Office of Education, *New Statistical Tables, Fiscal 1965.*

schools attests to this drive for self-improvement first and work later.

Still others are between the extremes; they want a certain amount of education—say, an A.A. or a B.A.—and within that time to specialize in a major field which they feel will lead to the best career opportunities. For these groups, allied health training must be seen as a choice between training for other occupations, and no training at all.

It is quite possible to work in many of the allied health occupations without having taken formal training. Fincher in Georgia and the Department of Labor in New York State found that a minority of jobs were held by professionally certified workers except where state licensure required it. Formal training may be necessary in the long run for a professional career, but in the short run the worker may profit more by foregoing training and entering directly into employment. Or, he might profit by foregoing the specialized training and follow a general education curriculum which would suit him not only for a health job but for a number of other jobs as well. For example, four years as a medical technology major in college prepares one only as a medical technologist, whereas a bachelor's degree in chemistry or biology enables one to enter upon any one of a large number of jobs, including medical technology. If a number of different training programs in the same occupation were available, the student might choose the best, or he might choose the shortest or the cheapest. Quality, duration, and expense are not necessarily directly correlated.

As mentioned before, many people will decide that they want a certain amount of education and will then look for the field which appears to offer the best investment for the future. Many health occupations suffer badly by comparison. The low wages, lack of advancement, and irregular hours in health work are so notorious that the recent improvements in many areas cannot overcome their poor reputation. Vocational-school and junior-college students who are considering their futures have alternatives that are much brighter or, what is more significant, they think they have.

Still other people, and possibly the majority, have no particular goal in mind and will take whatever happens to be readily available. Studies of job-seeking behavior among noncollege workers have uniformly shown that job seeking is not based so much on rational calculation as on chance, opportunity, and the influence of friends.[13] It could be argued that there is the same element of haphazardness in the choice of training programs. A number of persons might take training simply because it is there, or because one of their friends took it and liked it. The mere availability of low-cost training programs might influence the numbers of people entering health services.

One could question whether the 40,000 people trained in health services under MDTA would have entered health services or in any event would have sought training on their own had MDTA not been available. The chances are that they would not have, since the program is focused on the unemployed, underemployed, or disadvantaged who could not afford an investment in training. Training programs for lower-level workers are most successful when the student is paid for his efforts rather than having to pay. Such workers are not likely to have the resources to support themselves and perhaps their families for the duration of the program and are best able to take paid training, either through a training allowance as under MDTA, or through apprenticeship, on-the-job training, or company sponsored programs. (The "earn while you learn" slogan is most effective.) Similarly, the mere availability of training, even for

[13] Charles A. Myers and George P. Schultz, *Dynamics of a Local Labor Market* (New York, Prentice Hall, 1951), pp. 47–56; Lloyd G. Reynolds, *The Structure of Labor Markets* (New York, Harper, 1951), pp. 101–11; Harold L. Sheppard and A. Harvey Belltsky, *The Job Hunt: Job-Seeking Behavior of Uneducated Workers in a Local Economy* (Washington, Dept. of Labor, Office of Manpower Automation and Training, 1965).

those who are willing and able to pay for training or to support themselves while training, sometimes determines a person's future career. He will train for whatever occupation in which training is available. One cannot take advantage of an opportunity unless one knows it exists.

Other Influences on Choice

There are, of course, other important factors which influence a person's willingness or ability to take training in an allied health occupation. Among them are the cost of such training, an estimate of foregone income, knowledge of the existence of training programs, and geographic accessibility of the schools.

Despite recent efforts like the *Health Careers Guidebook* and the *Occupational Outlook Handbook* to disseminate information more broadly many health occupations are not well known. The United Hospital Fund of New York City recently asked a group of interested high-school guidance counselors about health careers. The results of one questionnaire follows:

Q. Do you feel you have sufficient information in your files on the following health careers to feel competent in counseling your students?

	Percent	
	Yes	*No*
Cytotechnologist	0	100
Inhalation Therapist	0	100
EEG and EKG Technician	1	99
Orthoptist	1	99
Audiologist and speech pathologist	8	92
Certified laboratory technologist	13	87
Rehabilitation therapist	13	87
House keeper	17	83
Dispensing optician	21	79
Osteopathic physician	24	76
Medical record librarian	25	75
Nutritionist	30	70

	Percent	
	Yes	*No*
Medical social worker	30	69
Hospital administrator	31	69
Medical librarian	31	69
Medical technologist	34	66
Podiatrist	35	65
Physical therapist	38	62
Optometrist	37	63
Dental laboratory technician	41	59
Nurse Aide and Orderly	41	59
X-ray technician	41	59
Occupational therapist	42	58
Medical secretary	45	55
Dietician	50	50
Dental assistant	51	49
Dental hygienist	54	46
Dentist	63	37
Licensed practical nurse	63	37
Physician	67	33
Registered professional nurse	73	27

Even if full allowance is made for the guidance counselors' being overconscientious in saying "no," this questionnaire still illustrates the lack of information available among the people responsible for guiding high-school graduates into careers.

Another consideration from the student side is the location of the school. There is a tendency at all levels of education for the student to take advantage of educational facilities located near his home.

From data in the Dental Students Register, 1965–66, of the American Dental Association, we found that in the twenty-seven states having schools for dental students, 76 percent remained in the state of origin for schooling, 12 percent moved to a contiguous state, and 12 percent moved to a noncontiguous state. In the thirty-two states having schools for dental hygiene students, 82 percent remained in the state of origin, 9 percent moved to a contiguous state, and 9 percent moved to a noncontiguous state.

A study of applicants for admission and students entering graduate schools of social work in 1961 found that 52 percent of the applicants came from the seven states containing 26 or almost half of such schools. These seven states included 5 of the 7 schools admitting 100 or more students. "It would appear that where educational opportunities in the field of social work are available, students in a given state make use of them." [14] The same apparently holds true for all occupations.

But geographic location is a two-edged sword. The schools must be located not only where the potential students are, but also where potential employment is. Voluntary geographic mobility cannot be depended on to distribute the workers from their place of schooling to the place of employment. It has been found that trained workers in every category tend to migrate to places of high wages and high employment,[15] that is, to the cities from the rural areas, to the North from the South and to California from the Prairie states. Yet it is precisely these areas—rural, South, prairie—that are most in need of health workers. There may be more potential students in Washington, D.C., but training them in Washington does not help the hospitals in rural Virginia, whereas training them in rural Virginia might enable them to find jobs in Washington, D.C. Voluntary mobility, or the lack of it, therefore, helps determine the training needs of a local area. An area which is the recipient of in-migration can get along with fewer schools than an area which suffers from out-migration.

Alaska, for example, had only one training program in 1964 in any health occupation, and that one was a school of practical nursing in Anchorage. Yet there were almost 2,000 full-time workers excluding attending physicians in Alaska's civilian hospitals in the same year. Nevada, with slightly more than 3,000 workers, had 2 schools of medical technology, 1 of professional nursing, 2 in X-ray

[14] Dept. of Health, Education, and Welfare, "Closing the Gap," p. 52.

[15] Seymour L. Wolfbein, *Employment and Unemployment in the United States* (Chicago, Science Research Associates, 1964).

technology, and 7 in practical nursing.[16] The difference is accounted for by the large numbers of trained people migrating to
Alaska, which enables that state to do without its own schools. The
1960 Census illustrates for instance that 79 percent of the 20 to 24
year old groups and 66 percent of the 25 to 29 age bracket did not
live in Alaska five years earlier.[17]

The question of population to be served is an important one in
setting up training programs. In a large city, a program to train 50
licensed practical nurses a year would hardly help alleviate a shortage; in a less populated rural area there might not be enough work
for 25. This is a problem for all training schemes, whether federal
or state, professional or vocational. As we have pointed out, area
vocational institutes and community colleges are most responsive to
local needs, as they consider it part of their mandate to provide
education and training for jobs in the local community. Most of
them insist on a local feasibility study, but the hiring institutions are
not always accurate in their calculation of needs. They will sometimes say they "need" more workers than they can actually afford
to hire. In addition, their need may be satisfied by a one-cycle program, whereas the training institutions cannot afford the expense
of instituting a program unless they can be assured a continuing
market for their graduates. The American Association of Junior
Colleges, for example, cautions its member colleges against setting
up expensive health curricula unless the continuing need for workers in an occupation will be enough to absorb an additional 15 or
20 workers every year over a long period of time.

Some Critical Problems

Allied health education and training has been subject to much criticism and controversy, not only from officials and administrators
within the field but from government officials, social scientists, and

[16] *Hospitals: Journal of the American Hospital Association,* Vol. 39, Part 2,
Guide Issue (August 1, 1965).
[17] *U.S. Census of Population,* PC (1) 3D.

the interested public. This concern with training derives, in large part, from the concern over quality of health care and even basic self-protection. Unlike goods-producing industries, the quality of the product of the health services industry is difficult, if not impossible, for the consumer to judge. When one cannot accurately judge the quality of the product, one attempts to gauge the quality of the producers. The quality most easily measured is education and training. It is, moreover, a quality that is to a large degree subject to external control. Thus, much of the concern for the quality of health care, and the attempt to improve it, turns into a concern for the quality of health care workers and an attempt to improve their education and training.

Two criticisms most often leveled against present health training are the lack of standardized quality in the various training programs for each occupation, and the lack of integration of training programs among the various occupations.

Lack of Standardization

Training for a given occupation varies among institutions. For one thing, occupational definitions vary from hospital to hospital. There is a lack of agreement on exactly what job tasks should be assigned to different groups of workers. [18] Each training institution has its own needs and desires which shape the training it gives. The variation in length of training discussed above is due to the differing educational philosophies of the respective institutions.

Standardized training for each occupation has several advantages and several disadvantages. One advantage is the ease of instituting a program. Without standardization, each institution has to start *de novo* with program planning—undoubtedly a large part of the initial costs. Another is the question of job mobility of trained workers. People trained for only one job in one institution will have

[18] Eugene Levine, Stanley Siegal, and Joseph De LaPuente, "Diversity of Nurse Staffing Among General Hospitals," *Hospitals,* Vol. 35 (1961), pp. 42–48; also Stephen J. Miller and W. D. Bryant, "How Minimal Can Nurse Staffing Be?" *The Modern Hospital* (October 1964).

difficulty transferring to another institution where the job may be slightly different, whereas people trained broadly for the occupation can adjust to a variety of particular jobs. A potential disadvantage is that standardization might lead to rigidity. Another is that the lowest standards may prevail.[19]

The greatest influence on standardization has come from the professional societies, which have attempted to raise the standards of health care by imposing standards of training. They have sometimes been assisted, and sometimes balked, by state laws demanding minimum qualifications for practice. State laws have the advantage of being enforceable, though they are not always enforced, but professional societies have the advantage of having nationwide influence. Recent efforts by the federal government to extend health training have also tended toward standardization, often by working with the relevant professional organization. The present project of the Hospital Research and Educational Trust provides standard training programs for low-skill-level occupations which have already been adopted in a number of hospitals.

One system of hospital care in which training is completely standardized is that of the Armed Forces. They retain centralized control over their hospitals and their staffs, and changes in staffing can be more easily integrated with changes in training procedures, a process impossible in the independent and uncoordinated civilian hospitals.

Lack of Integration

A second criticism leveled against the health training structure concerns the guild-like separation of occupations.[20] Training for each

---

[19] Ivar E. Berg, "Of Social Change and the Businessman," *Columbia Journal of World Business,* II (Summer 1966), 121–30.

[20] Dale L. Hiestand, "Research into Manpower for Health Services," National Institutes of Health, 1966; William Kissick, *Health Manpower in Transition* (Washington, Public Health Service, 1966); Lowell T. Coggeshall, *Progress and Paradox on the Medical Scene.*

occupation is complete in itself and based on the idea that the trainee has no previous knowledge or skills. Thus an experienced licensed practical nurse who wishes to become a registered nurse usually receives no credit for her skills. She must enter nurses' training on the same footing as an inexperienced untrained high-school graduate. The same holds true for different occupational levels in other health areas, and for occupations at the same level in different areas.

In general, as each new occupation arrives on the scene it develops its own training programs. Although there is much knowledge common to all, there is as yet little integration of basic education. Even the recent MDTA programs follow the tradition of training the worker only for the specific occupation. This is partly due to the influence of the professional societies—they do not wish to give up their hard-won independence. Not being too secure in their own status, they fear competition from lower-level personnel.

Most students are concerned that this lack of integration leads to overly rigid barriers on the job, and prevents, or makes difficult, the upward mobility of capable workers through the various levels. Coggeshall summarizes this position: "When persons working in a team share a common educational background, communication is facilitated and productivity increased. Perhaps the most significant shortcoming of the multiple tract system which precludes horizontal mobility is that it also precludes vertical mobility. We cannot interest the best people in the paramedical professions if these professions are dead-ends professionally, financially, and even socially." [21]

The argument in favor of integration of training for the various levels is obvious. It would enable workers to rise in the hierarchy by moving in and out of the educational system at various levels without having to return to the beginning each time. This might serve to increase the level of ability found among workers at the various strata. A job that is known to be a steppingstone to higher and bet-

[21] Coggeshall, *Progress and Paradox.*

ter jobs will attract highly able people, including some who cannot afford the initial outlay in time and money for the highest level of training. Conversely, recent experience with some governmental programs indicates that training will not be accepted by people who realize that the occupation is a dead-end one.

A possible disadvantage is that in any integrated system the highest profession will tend to predominate. Already much criticism is leveled at the AMA for dominating the medical field. It is also possible that a fully integrated system in each field might freeze out new occupations which are not presently part of the established fields.

The Armed Forces are often held up as a model in this regard. All health trainees are required to take a "core" course in basic health sciences before going into their specialization training, and each specialty proceeds in stages. For example, to become a dental technician a man must first take dental technician training, which qualifies him as a journeyman. However, he cannot go on from there to become a dentist. Workers in occupations requiring college degrees are generally recruited with all of their education completed.

Civilian hospitals sometimes promote occupational integration not by planning but by virtue of manpower shortages. It is often easier to assign a nurse's aide or a practical nurse as an assistant in a specialty than to train a new worker. It has been suggested that an expansion of existing practical nursing schools or nurse's-aide programs could be accomplished more easily than can the construction of new schools, and that this would produce people with a relatively broad basic training and a high degree of occupational transferability. But nursing training is itself a specialization and is not necessary for all workers. In addition, the identification of all levels of nursing with feminine work would deter many males from entering training.

There is a certain amount of coordination in the various training programs at present. The dental profession has long promoted training programs for dental hygienists and dental assistants. The medical technologists are fairly closely allied with the clinical pathologists. Recently, various health professions have begun to sponsor programs for lower-level assistants. But all of these lack the possibility for vertical or diagonal mobility.

A few steps have been taken toward integration along general lines. Some schools such as St. Mary's Junior College, the New York City Community College, and the College of Health Related Professions of the University of Florida have begun or are beginning to incorporate health curricula that include many specialties. The Allied Health Professions Personnel Training Act of 1966, which provides financial support for the construction of training facilities and the development of new curricula, is expected to increase the number of such schools (see Chapter 7).

A new California law for clinical laboratory personnel requires all laboratory technicians to have completed college and to take a state examination. After five years they are eligible to take the Clinical Bioanalyst licensing examination, which would entitle them to direct their own laboratories. These latter examinations are very difficult—70 percent fail—and in the future the prospective bioanalyst will be required to have an M.A. and eventually a Ph.D. But it does provide a career ladder and the possibility of advancement. New York City's new licensing law has similar provisions.

Present Position and Prospects

Training is inextricably meshed with employment. The concern for increasing the supply of health workers is co-joined with the desire to raise the quality of health service, and most of the latter efforts have been concentrated on increasing training levels.

Unquestionably, a large amount of allied health training does take place, mostly in hospitals, hospital-based schools, and colleges.

Nor is there any doubt that such training will increase as health employment increases, although not in lockstep. There is a tendency for programs to lag behind employment.

A clear trend is the increasing takeover of allied health training by colleges and junior colleges. This trend is accelerated by state and federal government programs aimed at the colleges, and also by increasing hospital costs, which render such training less feasible in hospitals.

To date, efforts to standardize the length, cost, and quality of the various types of training programs have been less than fully successful. The various and often conflicting needs and desires of the training institution, the students, and the employers cause problems in these matters.

On the whole, allied health training programs are not yet flooded with applicants. There is little knowledge of health occupations other than about doctors and nurses, and even less knowledge of training opportunities.[22] The informational efforts now being made by professional organizations and governmental agencies should serve to increase the awareness of health training and careers, although the well-earned reputation of the health services as offering poor job opportunities will probably continue to make such programs less popular than equivalent programs in other occupations.

---

[22] See, however, the recent booklet, *Horizons Unlimited,* published by the American Medical Association (1966), which covers a large spectrum of health occupations.

CHAPTER 5

Structure and Function of
Allied Health Labor Markets

IN DEALING WITH the labor force in the health services, we are not only confronted with one of the largest occupational complexes in the nation but also one of the most fragmented—"Balkanized," to use Clark Kerr's apt phrase. Among the reasons for the great deviations between the classical competitive model of a labor market and the medical one are the fact that hospitals, the major institutional employers, are largely in the not-for-profit sector; that occupational lines are more or less rigidly defined and constrained by legal and extra-legal restrictions; that the labor force is predominantly female; that unions have only recently become an important force; that a significant amount of work is performed by volunteers; and that the field as a whole is so vitally associated with the "public welfare."

It would be incorrect however, to infer from these caveats that market forces, such as wage incentives, for example, are less effective for health than for nonhealth manpower. What we wish to point out here is that the factors underlying the demand for and supply of labor in this area operate within a relatively large variety of institutional constraints and that these must be identified and analyzed if real and useful insights into the operation of allied health labor markets are to emerge.

It should be noted at the outset that there are almost as many labor markets as there are health occupations. The demand for nurse's aides, for example, is different from the demand for medical technologists although the demand for both is also influenced by general factors affecting the aggregate demand for medical care, or more specifically, the demand for personnel by hospitals. Kerr's description of an institutional labor market (as opposed to a "free choice" or "natural market") fits the situation of health labor markets very well: "Institutional rules in the labor market . . . establish more boundaries between labor markets and make them more specific and harder to cross. They define the points of competition, the groups which may compete and the grounds on which they compete." [1] In effect, the health labor market may be described as one of noncompeting groups of workers and, in some instances, the situation approaches that of a closed shop where membership in a professional association or group must precede employment.

To obtain a realistic view of the labor market situation, we attempt first to delineate those characteristics which distinguish the allied health from the general labor force. Next we examine the major changes that have taken place in the labor force from the employment, wage, and demographic aspects since 1950 using a fifteen-area sample of the United States. The chapter concludes with suggestions for making health labor markets more effective as allocative and distributive mechanisms within the context of the more efficient utilization of manpower and ultimately of the optimum delivery of health services.

Special Characteristics

In 1965 the total labor force of the United States (including the Armed Forces) numbered about 78.4 million. Of these, some 26.7

[1] Clark Kerr, "The Balkanization of Labor Markets," Reprint #59 (University of California, Institute of Labor Relations, 1954), p. 109.

million, or about 34 percent, were female.[2] In the area of health services, as was pointed out in Chapter 2, female workers constituted (as of 1960) 70 percent of the labor force and in hospitals in particular, where over two-thirds of all health workers are employed, 75 percent were women. In establishments other than hospitals (e.g., clinics, private offices of physicians and dentists, nursing homes, etc.) the female ratio decreased but women still constituted the majority of workers—60 percent in 1960. Moreover, in the decade of the 1950s, female workers in the health services rose by 67 percent compared with only a 32 percent increase for males.[3] (The sex ratios are analyzed in greater detail below.) Clearly, the labor force in health is predominantly a female one. The "core" or autonomous occupations within the health field however are almost entirely male, leaving the females dominant in the allied health categories. Apart from any other factors, this sex dichotomy is one explanation of the huge wage differences that are found among occupations in the medical field as a whole, and it is a major cause of the relatively high turnover rate among health personnel.

In terms of race, there are over twice the percentages of nonwhite females in health relative to all other industries (9 percent vs. 4 percent), but in the case of nonwhite males, there is a lower ratio in health than in industries in general (4 percent vs. 6 percent). However, when one looks at overall participation rates, both nonwhite males and nonwhite females slightly exceed their white counterparts, viz., 3 percent of all nonwhite males are employed in health services compared with 2 percent for whites and 9 percent of all nonwhite females are employed in health relative to 8 percent of white females. The two health occupations where the greatest concentration of nonwhite females is found are those of attendants (24

[2] *Manpower Report of the President, 1966,* Table A-1, p. 153.

[3] "Manpower in the 1960s," *Health Manpower Source Book,* Section 18 (Washington, Dept. of Health, Education, and Welfare, 1964), p. 5.

percent in 1960) and practical nurses and midwives (14 percent in 1960).[4]

The Nature of the Employing Firms

From a description of the sex and race features of the allied health employees we turn next to a consideration of the structure of the firms in which they are actually employed to see more clearly the relationship between the employing firms and the workers.

In Chapter 1 the economic aspects of the hospital as a facility for providing health services were analyzed and earlier in this section it was pointed out that over two-thirds of all health personnel are employed in hospitals. It is the latter aspect that interests us here, since historically the hospital has been and continues to be the focal point for the employment of medical personnel of all types. This dominant position also implies that its influence, so far as wages, hours, and working conditions are concerned, extends to other kinds of facilities where the remainder of the medical labor force is employed, an assertion which is reinforced by the consideration that the average number of employees per hospital was 294 (as of 1966), whereas the average number of people employed in nursing homes, private offices, and clinics and laboratories is far less—varying from one or two in private offices to a somewhat greater number in large laboratories and nursing homes, but in only relatively few cases does the employment total approach that of the average hospital.[5]

We must be alert, however, to the changes that are taking place in the health field. With the growing number of community health facilities—large prepaid closed or open panel groups, larger, more

[4] *Ibid.*, pp. 4 and 13.

[5] *Hospitals: Journal of the American Hospital Association,* Vol. 41, Part 2, *Guide Issue* (August 1, 1967), p. 452; "Technology and Manpower in the Health Service Industry, 1965–75," *Manpower Research Bulletin No. 14* (Washington, Dept. of Labor, May 1967), pp. 9, 10, and 11.

elaborate nursing homes and extended care facilities—and with the shift away from the hospitals and toward schools for basic educational functions, the ratio of hospital-based to total health workers is likely to decrease, and with it, the importance of the hospital as the chief determinant of wages, hours, and working conditions. Eventually, perhaps, the hospital may find itself in the position of a price (wage) taker rather than that of a price (wage) maker. Currently, however, the hospital may be viewed as the key bargainer and pattern-setter in the employment and earnings of workers in the health services industry—and it is also important to note that wages and salaries constitute the great bulk of total hospital expenses (roughly 60 to 70 percent at current levels).

Like other firms, hospitals vary by type, by size of plant, by geographic location, and by control (i.e., private, governmental, and not-for-profit or voluntary). For the purpose of the present analysis, it will be useful to conceive of a representative hospital—to borrow a term from Marshall—that is to say, a voluntary short-term general hospital with a complement of 150 to 200 beds and with about 300 employees. (For more specific analytic purposes one might wish to consider the separate labor problems presented by long-term general or psychiatric hospitals with larger bed complements and somewhat different labor mixes.)

The effects of the hospital on the labor market, and vice versa, stem from a variety of factors: the numbers employed, the occupational structure, the wage structure, the nature of the demand for workers (i.e., a basic complement with provisions for a 24-hour–7-day operation), relationships among workers in contiguous job families (e.g., varieties of nurses), the role of governments, professional organizations, and unions, the area from which workers can be drawn, budgetary considerations, competition from other health facilities, and ultimately from other industries.

To the labor market analyst, the hospital appears as a collection of independent craft guilds much the same as the separate crafts in the building construction industry. But whereas the specific *raison d'être* of the construction unions is collective bargaining on the issues of wages, hours, and working conditions, most of the medical and allied health associations do not consider the economic question to be their primary responsibility. The state nurses associations (not the American Nurses' Association) stand almost alone in this respect with their direct negotiation activities.

This is not to imply, of course, that these professional organizations have no interest in wages, rather, the attempt is made to influence wages indirectly—via licensing laws, minimum qualifications, and the like. Simon Rottenberg has pointed out several important economic consequences of such laws: they increase the cost of entry into the occupation; they generally produce favorable income effects for the licensees; they usually result in a higher age of entry into the trade; and usually, longer periods of schooling are required than are objectively necessary for the learning of the skills and knowledge relevant to the practice of the craft.[6] We should hasten to add, however, that not all of the professional groups are uniformly successful in achieving all of those objectives either directly or indirectly.

Typically, workers with the appropriate training and/or experience enter hospital employment by way of their particular specialty or subspecialty. The demand for the worker is usually initiated by a departmental head (laboratory, X-ray, dietary, etc.) and is communicated to the personnel department where, if the budget permits, the technicalities of screening and the completion of employment forms are accomplished.

This situation may be described as one of multiple ports of entry (each job is a separate port) and there is little mobility for the worker either in a vertical direction within a given occupation or in

[6] Simon Rottenberg, "The Economics of Occupational Licensing," in *Aspects of Labor Economics*, a conference of the Universities–National Bureau Committee for Economic Research (Princeton, Princeton University Press, 1962), pp. 4, 5, 14, and 19.

a horizontal direction, that is, between and among occupations. As one writer put it:

In no other industry is the "pecking order" more evident. From the viewpoint of a nurse's aide, no matter how experienced or capable she is, becoming an LPN is almost as remote as becoming a Ph. D. To become an LPN she must leave her job, which is impossible for the economically disadvantaged (the usual status for this nonprofessional occupation), and take a prescribed number of institutional training hours until she is deemed qualified in accordance with state law. She will be given no credit toward certification for her experience or capabilities. Even if she does get to be an LPN, and then aspires to become an RN, she will have to begin all over again. The institutional training necessary to become an LPN would be rendered worthless. All of this, in light of critical nurse shortages, defies any logic that can be brought to bear upon the situation.[7]

By contrast, many industries have fewer entry vestibules but once in, the worker finds relatively greater opportunities for internal (vertical or lateral) mobility. This well-deserved reputation of hospitals as repositories of dead-end occupations constitutes a serious impediment to recruitment as well as to continued attachment of workers to hospital employment. But we must guard against overdrawing this picture lest we lose touch with reality. Because of the combination, on the one hand, of Rottenberg's point of overeducation for jobs and, on the other, of the amount of learning that takes place on the job, considerable overlapping of functions occurs in the hospital, leading to jurisdictional disputes between contiguous groups such as the LPN and RN, the medical technicians and technologists, and even the RN and the MD. These interoccupational disputes, which may be expected to increase, not only are a source of friction among workers but are also the cause of a malutilization of hospital manpower. Too many manpower analyses have empha-

[7] Martin Karp, "OJT: Solution for Health Manpower Shortages," in *Employment Service Review*, Vol. 3, No. 11 (November 1966), p. 61.

sized the enormous skill differential in the hospital—say from a nurse's aid to neurosurgeon—and have not given sufficient attention to the overlapping functions or the connecting linkages of the occupations between the extremes.

Another important characteristic of the hospital, in its relation to the labor market, is the fact that it is all but completely immobile. In this respect, it may be compared to a steel mill, a shipyard, or a public school. Further, the usual criteria for industrial plant location such as wage rates, skill and resource availability, transportation accessibility, tax structure, and the like do not generally enter into the decision to locate in one area or another. (The growth of area-wide planning councils diminishes only slightly the force of this statement.) The implications in terms of the labor market of the fact that the hospital exists primarily to serve the local population (local has been extended to a "trading area" concept) are developed by Donald Yett, as follows:

Although there are over 7,000 hospitals in the U.S. the relevant labor market for each hospital is not so much national as local. And, on a local basis many hospitals are practically "monopsonists" (monopoly employers). For example, over 10 percent of all general hospitals are the only hospitals in their Hill-Burton service area; approximately 30 percent are in one-or-two hospital service areas; and over 40 percent are in areas with three or less hospitals. Under these circumstances, hospital administrators and personnel managers must be well aware of the futility of bidding against each other for the local supply of nurses.[8]

We might add that the occupation-specific nature of most allied health occupations tends to reinforce the monopsonistic power of the local hospital. There are few alternative industries which have a demand for more than a relative handful of general duty nurses. It should be pointed out, however, that while there may be little bidding up of wages, the competition for personnel takes other forms

[8] Donald E. Yett, "The Supply of Nurses: An Economist's View," *Hospital Progress* (February 1965), p. 100, n.18.

such as the provision (by subsidization usually) of well-appointed nurses' residences, more time off, tuition refunds, and other perquisites. Of course, the nurse may also opt to leave nursing altogether.

There are some additional structural and locational characteristics of the hospital as a locus of employment that bear on the allied health labor market:

1. Unlike firms or plants (in the private sector for the most part) which have well-defined managerial structures, hospitals are marked by diffuse control. The objectives of the medical staff, the administrative staff, and of the trustees are not conflict-free. This type of organization, where "nobody is in charge" is not conducive to efficient personnel management or, where unions may be involved, to efficient collective bargaining procedures.

2. Hospital beds tend to be concentrated in urban areas.[9] This means, among other things, that hospital wages will tend to be influenced in part by the general wage level of the city on the one hand, but it also means that there is greater opportunity for the hospital worker to seek employment in other hospitals (assuming no collusion on wages and the absence of gentleman's no-raiding agreements).

3. A corollary of the foregoing is the fact that an urban location is more attractive to most professional and paraprofessional personnel. This generates acute staffing problems for nonurban facilities.

4. The fact that the hospital must remain open twenty-four hours of every day makes work-scheduling a critical problem. Other institutions, however, such as telephone companies and police and fire departments are faced with and, to greater or lesser degrees, solve the same problem. Where the hospital differs from some of the other organizations is that in many cases the necessary kinds of physicians and surgeons, themselves not usually full-time employees of the hospital, may not be readily available. The trend to-

[9] *Manpower Report,* Table 5, p. 111.

ward the greater use of staff physicians, combined with appropriate use of shift differentials and "on call" pay for health personnel, should go far to even out the work load, thus contributing to over-all efficiency in manpower use.

5. Related to efficient work-scheduling as well as to general personnel shortages is the use of part-time workers. Contrary to what is commonly believed, the use of part-time workers in the medical and health services is not very great. As of 1965, 18 percent of workers who worked during that year worked at part-time jobs in health. While the ratio is high relative to the goods-producing sector, it is low relative to other industries in the services sector.[10] Of course, the ratio varies considerably by occupation. Generally more nurses work part-time than do other types of personnel. In any case there appears to be ample room for overcoming at least some of the health manpower shortages by the use of more part-time workers.

Labor Market Developments

We turn next to the empirical data—to what has actually happened in the market for allied health personnel in recent years with respect to the basic questions of employment and earnings.

National Employment Changes

The gross picture of long-term employment changes of health manpower which was provided in Chapters 1 and 2 must be supplemented by a variety of other types of data to obtain a fuller understanding of allied health labor market developments. The data

[10] "Work Experience of the Population in 1965," *Special Labor Force Report No. 76,* Table A-2, pp. A7–A8. *Monthly Labor Review Reprint* (December 1966). In a recent Washington state survey of 15 medical occupations listing vacancies, only one—dental hygienist—showed any vacancies for part-time employment. See "Occupational Trends in Health Care Industries, King County, 1965–1970" (State of Washington, Dept. of Employment Security and State Board for Vocational Education, December 1965), Table 3, p. 5.

to be presented in the remainder of this section accordingly will deal with different time periods, with regional and area changes, with demographic factors, as well as with more detailed occupational groups.

The first point to be made in connection with aggregate medical employment is that the strong growth trend evident between 1950 and 1960 and earlier has persisted into the 1960s. As the data in Table 5.1 show, nonagricultural employment in the United States increased by 14 percent between 1959 and 1965, whereas employment in medical and health services rose by 44 percent—more than three times as fast. Employment in each of the subgroups shown also rose by considerably higher rates than did the nonagricultural sector, with one group—"Other Medical Services"—having increased at a rate which was more than five times the aggregate figure. (Included in this group are medical and dental laboratories, group health facilities, sanitoria, and convalescent and rest homes).

Table 5.1

Employment Changes, Total Nonagricultural and Health Services, 1959–1965

	1959	1965	Percent
	(*in millions*)		*Change*
Total nonagricultural employment	53.3	60.8	+14
Medical and other health services *	1.453	2.087	+44
Hospitals	.967	1.364	+41
Offices of Physicians and Surgeons	.207	.280	+36
Offices of Dentists and Dental Surgeons	.080	.105	+31
Other †	.183	.318	+73

* Medical categories taken from Standard Industrial Classification code.
† As of March of the stated year.
Source: "Employment and Earnings Statistics for the United States, 1909–1966," *Bureau of Labor Statistics Bulletin No. 1312-4*, pp. xvi, 690–91, and 778.

Regional Employment and Earning Changes

It is one of the working hypotheses of this book that the strong and persistent increases in employment of all types of health manpower—especially at the non-core (or if one prefers, outer-core) levels—arises basically from increases in the aggregate effective demand for health services, with changing technology playing an important but subordinate role. An examination of wage trends is undertaken here to help arrive at a judgment as to whether the demand for services has, in fact, increased at a greater rate than the supply of workers. If this has been the case then we might also examine the data for signs of the classic techniques used by employers to adjust to the conditions of labor shortage. Richard Lester has identified the most important of these as: changes in recruitment methods; lowering quality standards for new employees; special increases in starting rates, maintenance rates, or hiring of new employees above starting rates or into higher than normal job classes; changes in production methods; and substituting female or part-time workers—to which we would add ethnic minorities, and in the medical occupations, substitution of male for predominantly female workers.[11] Changes in production methods have already been commented on in Chapter 1. The data which follow will shed some light on the other points.

Generally, labor shortages are not confined to a single employer. More often they affect groups of employers and entire areas. Furthermore, any attempts to deal with shortages usually channel through a political unit with responsibility for a given geographical area be it federal, state, or municipal. Consequently analyses which purport to have an influence on policy must be oriented toward regional variations and problems. The following analysis therefore attempts to take such regional factors into account.

[11] Richard I. Lester, "Adjustments to Labor Shortages" (Princeton University, Dept. of Economics and Sociology, Industrial Relations Section, 1955).

Table 5.2, based on 1950 and 1960 Census data, sets out the decadal changes in nonagricultural employment, in employment of hospital personnel, and in what might be termed the basic hospital manpower endowment of fifteen major standard metropolitan statistical areas (SMSA) of the United States for 1950 and 1960. These areas represent (though they may not be completely representative of) all of the major regions of the country and all but one (Mountain) of the subregions.

Table 5.2

Changes in Nonagricultural and Hospital Employment in Selected Areas, 1950 to 1960

Standard Metropolitan Statistical Area	Percent Change in Employment		Total Population ÷ Hospital Employment	
	Nonagri- cultural	Hospital	1950	1960
Atlanta	38	54	160	146
Baltimore	18	56	105	83
Boston	13	32	87	71
Buffalo	14	74	124	86
Chicago	13	49	171	140
Cincinnati	18	57	123	93
Cleveland	16	55	111	87
Dallas	45	133	296	185
Los Angeles– Long Beach	49	91	188	157
Memphis	22	39	78	73
Minneapolis–St. Paul	23	60	89	72
New York City	12	48	107	81
Philadelphia	16	53	127	98
Portland	17	43	111	90
San Francisco	23	56	154	137

The major point to note is that the aggregate national experience with respect to the relatively greater increases in health manpower that was previously documented is repeated in each of the fifteen areas. In each area, increases in employment of hospital personnel far exceeded increases in nonagricultural employment over the decade of the 1950s. (Allowance should, of course, be made for the different base magnitudes.) The second point of interest is the great inter-area variation in hospital manpower endowment, here measured by the ratio of population to hospital personnel. In 1950, for example, the Dallas area stood out as the least endowed in terms of this index, and the Memphis area as the best endowed. Ten years later, every one of the fifteen areas showed an improvement with respect to this measure, with Dallas retaining its rank on the list and Boston moving to the "best endowed" position. For the group as a whole, whereas in 1950, twelve of the fifteen areas had population-manpower ratios of over 100, in 1960, the number of such areas was reduced to five.

The last two censuses enable us to determine for seven major health occupations first, what the male–female ratios were, and second, whether there was any change in these ratios between 1950 and 1960. An examination of these data indicated few substantial changes in the sex ratios. As might be expected, professional and practical nurses showed female ratios of well over 90 percent in both periods, with little interperiod change. Pharmacists, traditionally a male group, remained so between 1950 and 1960. The high female ratio in the medical and dental technician group became even higher in 1960 relative to 1950. There were some interesting changes in the sex composition of hospital and institutional attendants. In 1950, females constituted a minority of this group in only two areas: Atlanta (37.2 percent) and Memphis (44.9 percent). By 1960, there was a marked change in both cases; in Atlanta, the ratio increased to 68.2, and in Memphis to 62.7. This may be a reflection of the fact that better opportunities became available for males, both white and Negro, during this period.

Turning to the racial composition in these same occupations for 1950 and 1960, we find that the nonwhite ratio increased in each one of the seven occupations under review. In the case of medical and dental technicians and professional nurses, the nonwhite ratio increased in each of the fifteen areas; dieticians, hospital attendants, and practical nurses showed increases in the nonwhite ratio in fourteen areas; the ratio for pharmacists increased in twelve areas; and that for therapists and healers in ten areas.

From these data it appears that the racial barriers have been easier to pierce than were those related to sex. This would seem to imply two things: that even in occupations with relatively high growth rates, strong taboos persist with respect to male employment —nurses for instance; the second implication—and this is one on which subsequent data may bear—is that the wage rates were still too low to attract males, especially those with family responsibilities.

Some prefatory remarks concerning the general hospital wage situation are in order before we examine its structural and regional aspects. The hospital as an employing organization, to a large extent, has been insulated from the labor market pressures that normally act on firms in the private sector, and even on some in the not-for-profit sector. We can identify several reasons for this. First, the hospital provides services mainly on a local basis, therefore it is generally considered to be intrastate in character. As such, it did not fall automatically under the jurisdiction of federal legislation such as the Fair Labor Standards Act. Only recently (1966) was the FLSA amended to cover hospital workers. The new amendments, which became effective February 1, 1967, provided for a minimum hourly wage for hospital and nursing home workers of $1.00, rising in four steps to $1.60 in 1971. It was correctly observed, however, that : "In its present form, provisions of the legislation will have only moderate effects in the short run on existing pay differentials between employment in hospitals and nursing homes and other industries; for under the same new law, minimum wage levels for workers already covered became $1.40 on February

1, 1967 and will step up to $1.60 on February 1, 1968. Substantial differences between the earnings of health service workers and workers in non-health jobs will continue for a long while." [12] Second, hospitals are primarily nonprofit (voluntary) institutions—in 1965, for example, 70 percent of all hospital beds were under this type of control. Consequently, hospitals were generally exempt from state minimum wage laws as well as from other types of labor legislation such as unemployment insurance. Third, since so large a proportion of hospital jobs are specific and nontransferable, the hospital has an advantage over the worker who finds it difficult to secure nonhospital employment. Fourth, the hospital, more so than any other institution, has had the good fortune of filling a not inconsiderable number of jobs with volunteer workers. Fifth, the hospital has been relatively free from wage pressures exerted by unions. In fact, one of the largest groups of hospital workers, the professional nurses, reinforced this lack of pressure by adopting a no-strike policy in 1950. [13] (There has been a vigorous movement of late to have that policy altered.) Estimates of the percent of hospital workers unionized vary from a low of about 5 percent to a high of about 15 percent.[14] In any case, hospitals would rank at or near the bottom of the scale as far as unionization is concerned, but this is an area which appears to be changing rapidly.[15]

To these rather concrete factors might be added another which lies in the subjective area, namely, hospital workers themselves may feel that even though they may be relatively underpaid, the character of their work—service to patients—adds a nonpecuniary incre-

[12] "Technology and Manpower," p. 17.

[13] "Major Official Policies Relating to the Economic Security Program," *Publication No. EC-10* (New York, American Nurses' Association, 1965), p. 3.

[14] "Technology and Manpower," p. 17, in addition to a personal interview with officials of hospital unions.

[15] For a useful overview of hospital–union problems, see Estelle Hepton, "Battle for the Hospitals: A Study of Unionization in Nonprofit Hospitals," *Bulletin No. 49* (Ithaca, Cornell University, New York State School of Industrial and Labor Relations, March, 1963).

ment to their actual earnings. Workers in steel mills or in machine tool factories are less likely to indulge in similar calculations. The ensuing data, though they may not bear directly on all of the factors just mentioned, should nevertheless be viewed against that general backdrop.

Unfortunately, we do not have detailed wage data for medical occupations for 1950 so that we cannot make the wage comparisons for the 1950s that we were able to make for employment. There do exist, however, detailed wage data for 1956 so that at least one may get a picture of wage changes since that date.

A Bureau of Labor Statistics survey of hospital wages showed that between 1956 and 1960, the median city increase in average earnings in each of 11 occupations (ranging from supervisors of nurses to nurse's aides) exceeded the increase in average earnings in manufacturing during the same period. The latter increase was 14 percent compared with a 24 percent increase for dieticians, a 23 percent increase for nurse supervisors and 23 and 22 percent increases for medical technologists and medical record librarians respectively.[16] This is presumptive evidence, at least, of some tightness in the medical labor market over this period. Of course, there is no contradiction between these data and the fact that, in 1962, for example, the average yearly compensation of health service workers was still below the average for all employees, $3,435 and $5,449 respectively.[17] The question here is whether and how fast that gap is closing.

A recent study of this matter by the Associated Hospital Service of New York (Blue Cross) indicated that average weekly salaries in manufacturing industries in New York City in 1960 were $84.36, but that they were $69.20 in the accredited voluntary general hospitals—a 22 percent differential. By mid-1965, both salary

[16] "Earnings and Supplementary Benefits in Hospitals, Mid-1960," *Bureau of Labor Statistics Bulletin No. 1294,* p. 5; and "Employment and Earnings Statistics for the United States, 1909–1966," *Bureau of Labor Statistics Bulletin No. 1312-4.*
[17] "Technology and Manpower," p. 15.

levels were equal at about $100 a week, and by the beginning of 1966 the hospital salaries slightly exceeded those in manufacturing —$104.87 to $101.95, a differential in favor of the hospital of 3 percent.[18]

As pointed out, a major focus of this chapter is the examination of area and regional changes with respect to health manpower and wage adjustments. Geographic wage differences for the same or similar occupations may be ascribed to several factors: differences in living costs; the presence or absence of unions and the degree of unionization; different supply–demand relationships; and different laws.

In the health occupations, as we have already seen, unions and legislation play minor roles. Generally, the difference in living costs may also be ignored when we are dealing with large cities or areas, for it has been observed that although individual cost-of-living items such as food and housing vary among cities, the variations in total living costs in metropolitan areas are not very great. We are led therefore to different supply–demand relationships as the major determinant of area wage differentials.

In attempting to arrive at some judgments regarding the supply and demand for labor in the different areas of our sample and specifically to determine whether wages in the health areas conform to general wage pressures, we ranked the areas by average earnings both in manufacturing and in several health occupations for the year 1960.[19] This study revealed a high degree of consistency between areas which ranked high in manufacturing earnings and those in medical earnings. The San Francisco area, for instance, which ranked highest in manufacturing, also placed in the top three earnings ranks of the seven occupations listed. At the other extreme, Dallas, which ranked lowest in manufacturing, also ranked

[18] J. Douglas Colman, "An Analysis of the Components of Rising Hospital Costs," *Blue Cross Reports,* Vol. V, No. 3 (August–September 1967).

[19] "Employment and Earnings Statistics for States and Areas, 1939–1965," *Bureau of Labor Statistics Bulletin No. 1370-3* and *No. 1294.*

low in all of the medical occupations with the exception of medical technologists, where it ranked sixth. Atlanta and Memphis were consistently low in both manufacturing and medical earnings, and San Francisco and Los Angeles were consistently high. There were some interesting inconsistencies as well: Boston ranked twelfth in manufacturing but fifth in practical nurse earnings; Buffalo was second in manufacturing and ninth in general duty nurse earnings; Cleveland was third in manufacturing but tenth in medical technologist earnings.

When selected earnings data are combined into a larger regional context, they provide still additional insights. The Western region, for example, exceeded all of the other regions in twelve of the fifteen cases. It is interesting to note, however, that for physical therapists, the South exceeded the Northeast in each of the three rates and exceeded the West in two of the three cases. When earnings in a generally low-wage area such as this exceed those in high-wage areas, a regional manpower deficit in the specific occupation in question may be inferred with some degree of confidence.

Publication by the Bureau of Labor Statistics of its series, *Earnings and Supplementary Benefits in Hospitals* (as of July 1966), permits some comparisons of medical earnings on our fifteen-area sample for the last full decade for which data are available, namely 1956–66.

For this period, we attempt to determine whether wage changes in medical occupations have been greater than nonmedical wage changes; what the differences are among areas as far as wage changes are concerned; whether inter-area differentials have become more uniform; and whether employment has been responsive both to the absolute as well as to the inter-area wage changes.

Here again we use as a base of reference the change in weekly earnings in manufacturing, which between 1956 and 1966 was 42 percent. Apart from the absolute levels of the wages and of the interoccupational differentials (not shown here)—which are of interest in their own right—the following summary points up some interesting relationships.

The first point that is impressive is the fact that, with relatively few exceptions, all of the medical occupations shown recorded wage increases in excess of those in manufacturing. Second, where wage changes of the magnitude recorded occurred in all of the areas,

Occupation	*Areas Where Wage Increases Equaled or Exceeded Manufacturing Wage Increases, 1956–1966*
Director of nursing	All but Dallas
Supervisor of nursing	All
Head nurse	All but Dallas
General duty nurse	All but Portland
Nursing instructor	All
Chief X-ray technician (male)	All but Cleveland and Baltimore
X-ray technician (male)	All but Philadelphia, Minneapolis–St. Paul, San Francisco–Oakland, and Portland
Medical technician (male)	All but Cleveland
Chief X-ray	All
X-ray technician	All but Dallas, Philadelphia, and Portland
Medical technician	All
Medical records librarian	All but Dallas and Cincinatti
Medical social worker	All
Physical therapist	All but Minneapolis–St. Paul
Dietician	All but Minneapolis–St. Paul
Practical nurse	All but Minneapolis–St. Paul
Nurse's aide (male)	All but Minneapolis–St. Paul, San Francisco–Oakland, and Chicago
Nurse's aide	All but Minneapolis–St. Paul

there is sound presumptive evidence of rather strong demand, nationwide, for these occupations. Third, since the same areas do not appear on the shortfall list (i.e., increase below those in manufacturing) for all occupations, we have a surrogate index of the relative manpower endowment in the various regions. Fourth, we can fairly easily identify those occupations which are in extremely short supply in the given areas by focusing on the wage increases, which, at a minimum, were twice as great as those in manufacturing. (For simplicity we use the 80 percent cut off instead of the technically correct 84 percent.) The results are as follows:

Wage Increases	*Area*
100 percent or more	Philadelphia, Los Angeles–Long
Medical social worker	Beach, Baltimore
Between 80 and 100 percent	New York City, Baltimore
Director of nursing	Baltimore
Supervisor of nursing	Baltimore, Boston
Head nurse	New York City
Nursing instructor	San Francisco–Oakland
Medical technologist	New York City
Chief X-ray technician	New York City
Medical records librarian	Baltimore
Physical therapist	Philadelphia
Practical Nurse	New York City
Nurse's aide (male)	New York City, Buffalo, Baltimore,
Nurse's aide	Philadelphia

With the exception of the nurse's aides and practical nurses, the other occupations in the 80 to 100 percent range are all at relatively higher levels on the occupational ladder. In the former case, part of the reason for the larger wage increases might be attributed to a catching-up process, but surely, a large part may be presumed to reflect the increased demand for these workers.

We examine next inter-area and intra-area changes in terms both of absolute wage levels and of interoccupational wage differentials. The purpose of these analyses is to shed some light on changes in the occupational and regional distribution of medical manpower in so far as these may have been responsive to and affected by wage pressures. An important question in this respect is whether regional wage variations for the same occupation are becoming more uniform or more dispersed over time. If the former is true then it might be assumed that medical personnel are becoming more evenly distributed among the regions; and if the latter, that the distribution is less even—a fact which in turn may be indicative of a drawing off of personnel from the lower to the higher wage area. Alternatively, these data may also reveal the disproportionate growth of existing hospitals in the various regions and/or the establishment of new hospitals and consequently of new demands for personnel. Supplementary data on hospital beds and on hospital visits (both inpatient and out) per area population for each of the SMSA's in our sample would shed additional light on this question. As of now, however, these data are not available.

Our first approach then is, within one area, to arrange the data in descending order, viz., from the most highly paid to the least paid of the major medical occupations in the BLS survey. From this array, we can, at a glance, see where a particular occupation stands in the wage hierarchy. By means of an intertemporal analysis we can also determine which occupations gained and which lost in relative position in the wage structure in this area from 1956 to 1966.

Let us look at one of the regions, New York City, for an illustration of the wage structure of hospital personnel and how that picture has changed over the ten-year period. This technique can provide a measure of the relative needs for various personnel in the regions covered by the survey. Table 5.3 presents the data in this form. It may be noted first that the difference between the highest salaried occupation (director of nursing: $112.50) and the lowest (female nurse's aide: $35.00) was $77.50. Of greater importance were the job categories (and these were the jobs which have large numbers of employees) below $40 per week in 1956 (the federal minimum wage at that time was $1.00 per hour). Over the next ten years there were large wage increases, and the difference between the highest salary ($206.50, again for director of nursing) and the lowest ($69.50, again for nurse's aide) increased to $137.00. We might note that in 1966 none of the jobs was below the minimum, which at $1.25 per hour for a 40-hour week would have been $50.00. Within the wage hierarchy there were also changes: social workers went down in rank from fourth to sixth, and female medical technologists rose in rank from sixteenth to thirteenth. The spread between the highest and lowest salaries increased in each of the fifteen areas studied. This resulted from the fact that while the increases at the lower end of the scale were usually (but not always) higher than those at the upper, there were large differences in the base figures themselves.

Table 5.3

Wages and Relative Rank of Selected Health Occupations, New York City, 1956 and 1966

1956		*1966*	
(1) Director of Nursing	$112.50	(1) Director of nursing	$206.50
(2) Chief X-ray technician (male)	102.50	(2) Nursing instructor	155.00
		(3) Chief X-ray technician	153.00
(3) Supervisor of nurses	86.00	(4) Supervisor of nurses	150.50
(4) Medical social worker	86.00	(5) Medical records librarian	150.50
(5) Medical records librarian	83.50	(6) Medical social worker	149.00
(6) Nursing instructor	82.50	(7) Chief X-ray technician (male)	145.50
(7) Chief X-ray technician	81.50		
(8) Head nurse	74.00	(8) Head nurse	132.00
(9) Dietician	72.00	(9) Physical therapist	125.50
(10) Physical therapist	70.00	(10) Dietician	124.00
(11) Housekeeper, chief	70.00	(11) Housekeeper, chief	120.50
(12) General duty nurse	67.50	(12) General duty nurse	119.50
(13) X-ray technologist (male)	66.50	(13) Medical technologist	113.00
(14) X-ray technologist	66.00	(14) X-ray technologist	111.00
(15) Medical technologist (male)	65.50	(15) X-ray technologist (male)	110.50
(16) Medical technologist	65.00	(16) Medical technologist (male)	108.00
(17) Practical nurse (male)	52.50	(17) Practical nurse	89.00
(18) Practical nurse	51.50	(18) Practical nurse (male)	87.00
(19) Nurse's aide (male)	39.00	(19) Nurse's aide (male)	72.50
(20) Nurse's aide	35.00	(20) Nurse's aide	69.50

Note: number in parentheses denotes rank.

Source: *BLS Bulletin No. 1254* and "Earnings and Supplementary Benefits in Hospitals," Area Release, New York City, July 1966.

An examination of the intra-area wage changes over the 1956–66 decade reveals those occupations which increased in relative rank, those which decreased, and those which remained constant. An increase in relative rank is presumed to indicate a relative shortage in the area and, a decrease in relative rank is indicative of a relative surplus. Relative rank increases occurred in many areas in the following occupations: head nurse, general duty nurse, female medical technician, medical social worker, dietician, physical therapist. Decreases in relative rank were pronounced for both male and female X-ray technican, and medical record librarian. The case of the female X-ray technicians is interesting. There was not one area where the rank increased. An obvious explanation would be that, for some unknown reasons, male X-ray technicians are in greater demand than female ones. This hypothesis is not supported, however, by a look at the male X-ray technician situation. While we found an increase in relative rank in two areas, the general picture of relative decreases prevailed. Moreover, the absolute increases in wages from 1956–66 for both groups were not significantly different. The only conclusions one can draw from these facts are: the supply of X-ray technicians is rather uniform over the areas in question; there does not appear to be a general shortage of X-ray technicians at least over the past ten years. The increased use of X-rays on patients appears to have been accomplished without a great increase in demand for technicians. Implicit in this hypothesis, however, is the assumption that the productivity of X-ray technicians has increased significantly without concomitant increases in wages.

The medical technologist groups showed almost the reverse pattern. There was only one area where this group lost in relative rank. In every other area it either remained unchanged or, more usually (ten areas), increased in rank.

It is important to emphasize that "unchanged" does not mean that the demand had not increased or that wages have not increased. We are discussing relative changes in wage hierarchy. Of course, it is not to be expected that nurse's aides, for example, who are the least skilled, and who occupy the bottom rung of the wage ladder, will change relative to the occupations which require somewhat greater minimum education or training. Moreover, this analysis does not reveal the extent to which employees of a given job family are actually doing the work of those whose titles, at least, place them on higher rungs.

So much for intra-area changes; we focus next on the inter-area ones.

Our analysis was designed to show the percentage wage differentials between regions for a given occupation. To illustrate: the highest average weekly wage for director of nursing in 1956 was found in the Minneapolis–St. Paul area. That rate was 2.9 percent greater than that which directors of nursing received in the next lower area, San Francisco–Oakland, which in turn exceeded the next lower rate in Chicago, by 1.7 percent, and so on. The wage difference between the highest and lowest regions for this occupation was 23 percent in 1956. Ten years later, this differential increased to 43.6 percent. Increases in aggregate regional wage differentials of this type may be indicative of several things: the desire of some areas (essentially the combined demands of the area hospitals) to attract personnel of a specific type from other areas by the inducement of higher wages and/or increases in wages arising from purely internal causes. However, even if the wage increase arose from purely endogenous factors, it still affects the area's relative standing, and it is this aspect which is under scrutiny here. We may point out that of the 14 medical occupations, regional differentials increased in 9, remained constant in 1, and decreased in 4. A decrease implies that the areas have become more homogeneous with respect to wage differences.

What strikes one immediately about this analysis is the overall uniformity it revealed. In the vast majority of cases, the wage differences between one region and the next lower one were less than 5 percent in order of magnitude. There were, however, a number of cases where the disparities were much greater. Examples: a 10 percent differential between the San Francisco–Oakland and Los Angeles–Long Beach areas for directors of nursing; a 17.2 percent differential between Buffalo and Dallas also for nursing directors; a 12 percent margin between San Francisco–Oakland and Chicago, and an 11 percent difference between New York City and Boston in medical record librarian wages; 18.5 percent between Los Angeles–Long Beach and Cincinnati for medical technologists; 13.8 percent between San Francisco–Oakland and Minneapolis for female nurse's aides; 14.8 percent between Minneapolis and Philadelphia in 1956 for female chief X-ray technicians.

An examination of these data also reveal that the top areas in terms of wages are San Francisco–Oakland, Minneapolis–St. Paul, Los Angeles–Long Beach, Cincinnati, and New York. The lowest regions generally were Baltimore, Memphis, Atlanta, Philadelphia, and Dallas. Of twenty-eight possibilities, Philadelphia appears at the bottom twelve times, Atlanta five, and Dallas three times.

Two hypotheses which suggest themselves to explain narrow inter-area differentials in a given occupation are that the distribution of personnel is fairly uniform and that some professional organization has succeeded in establishing national norms for its members. On the other hand, wider wage differentials may be indicative of shortages of specific occupations in some areas or they may be due to some special activities such as successful unionization drives or legislation (state minimum wage laws) which affect the area wage structure.

Even though the aggregate percentage wage difference between the high and low regions may have increased between 1956 and 1966, suggesting greater regional variance, closer inspection reveals that in 1966, most of the wage differences among the areas were concentrated in the 0 to 2 percent range, whereas in 1956, the range of differentials was wider. In 1966, nurse's aide was the only occupation which exhibited frequent wage differentials greater than the 0 to 2 percent range, indicating that there was still considerable inter-area diversity in the distribution of such personnel.

Nonregional Factors in Wage Differentials

Male–Female Differentials

Table 5.4 presents data on the percentages by which male wages exceeded female wages for the same occupation, again using our fifteen-area sample. This analysis indicates that there are distinct preferences for male over female workers in the following occupations: chief X-ray technicians, X-ray technologists, physical therapists, and nurse's aides. There was no clear sex preference in the case of medical technologists and practical nurses.

Registered vs. Nonregistered Personnel Differentials

An important source of wage differentials not revealed so far by the data is the question of registration or certification of the medical personnel we have been reviewing. There is, unfortunately, no indication in the BLS surveys as to whether the personnel (excluding the registered professional nurse) had achieved certain educational and training levels and had been certified by one of the professional groups or by the state as a registered X-ray technician, technologist, or whatever. If the wage data presented are averages, then they conceal the great amount of variation between registered and nonregistered differentials.

From a mail survey of our own of hospital wages, as reported by state hospital associations, we have derived data (Table 5.5) for a small sample of states and cities on wage differentials of registered vs. nonregistered technical medical personnel. We found that in every case the wage rates of registered exceeded those of nonregistered personnel, with the most usual differential falling between 20 and 30 percent.

Table 5.4

Male–Female Wage Differentials *
in Selected Health Occupations, 1956 and 1966

	Chief X-ray Technician		X-ray Technician		Medical Technician		Physical Therapist		Nurse's Aide		Practical Nurse	
	1956	1966	1956	1966	1956	1966	1956	1966	1956	1966	1956	1966
Atlanta				+23.1		−5.0				+9.0		
Baltimore		+15.2	−1.8	+9.4		−0.45			+11.4	−2.7		
Boston	+14.2	+21.2	−7.5	+6.8	+10.9	−0.49			+12.2	+4.5	−9.0	−11.6
Buffalo			+10.1	+10.4	+0.74	+4.7		+11.2	+24.4	+7.8		
Chicago	+1.7	+3.9	+4.8	+6.0	+6.0	+4.8		+24.1	+8.6	+5.4	+3.8	+9.9
Cincinnati				+1.1					+16.5	+9.1		
Cleveland			+9.0	+5.7	+9.5	+0.48		+7.4	+19.6	+13.8		
Dallas			−8.0	+2.7		+15.6			+22.4	+17.6		
Los Angeles–Long Beach		+3.6	+3.3	+1.4	0	−2.6		−2.3	+7.8	+6.7	+7.9	+6.7
Memphis				−0.57								
Minneapolis–St. Paul	+21.6	+12.8	+4.9	+1.8	+0.76	−4.6		+20.7	+7.1	+3.4		
New York City	+20.5	−5.2	+0.75	−0.45	+0.76	−4.6		+6.3	+10.3	+4.1	+1.9	−2.3
Philadelphia		+42.6	+0.88	−1.3	+8.9	+13.8		−6.2	+14.1	+0.91	+20.2	
Portland			−2.8	−0.50	+1.4	+1.3			+10.8	+5.4		
San Francisco–Oakland	+14.1	+10.7	+10.4	+1.3	+1.8	+3.7			+8.1	+2.3		

* Differential $= \dfrac{W_M - W_F}{W_M}$, where W_M = male wage, W_F = female wage.

Source: Same as Table 5.3.

Table 5.5

Wage Differentials: Registered–Nonregistered Health Personnel, in Selected Areas, 1965 and 1966
(in percent)

State or City	Medical Records Librarian	X-ray Technician	Medical Technician
Arizona (median)	35	22	25
Tucson (median)	74		12
Phoenix (median)	23	20	23
Missouri (median starting)	74	28	29
Maine (average starting)		16	16
Michigan (average going)		23	20
Wisconsin			
Milwaukee (mode)	29	3	1
			21 ASCP-MT
Madison (mode)	44	3	1
			32 ASCP-MT
Illinois (average)	40		19
			24 ASCP-MT
Chicago (average)	24		9
			33 ASCP-MT
Indiana (average going)	57	28	32
Virginia (average minimum)		20	28
Colorado			
Denver (starting)	24	12	27

Note: ASCP = American Society of Clinical Pathologists; MT = Medical Technologist

Source: Various reports from state hospital associations, 1965–66.

Wage rates of ASCP registrants exceeded nonregistered rates by amounts varying from a low of 12 percent in Tucson to a high of 33 percent in Chicago, with the most common differential once again falling in the same range as the first two cases, viz., 20 to 30 percent. The lower level medical technicians showed wage differences commonly on the order of 1 to 10 percent above nonregistered personnel, but wage deficits on the order of 20 to 30 percent relative to the ASCP people.

The important question here is whether the hospital specifies that registration be a condition of employment. Of course, where state legislation exists making registration of certain personnel mandatory, e.g., physicians, dentists, nurses (and recently, X-ray technicians in New York State), the hospital has no choice but to comply. But we should not underestimate, as one economist put it, "the strong economic leverage of a tight labor market." [20] In the absence of legislation, the personnel administrator may accept nonregistered personnel (who may nevertheless be fully qualified) and even where legislation exists, new occupational titles may be developed (e.g., operating room technician, inhalation therapist)—a procedure which, in effect, allows nonregistered personnel to perform functions that, according to the law, may only be performed by those who are certified. Finally, there are many cases where, under conditions of acute labor market tightness, the laws are honored more in their breach than in their observance. In any case, data collection agencies should be more sensitive to these problems and attempt to elicit information with respect to registration in future surveys.

Differentials by Control, Size of Place, and Size of Hospital

Another factor in the wage differentials of hospital personnel is associated with the hospital control type, that is to say, whether the hospital is owned or operated by governmental authorities, nonprofit associations, or proprietary groups. In the 1960, 1963, and 1966 surveys, the Bureau of Labor Statistics found that, generally, average salaries for most occupations were higher in government than in private hospitals. This is undoubtedly due to the fact that civil service wage scales are more likely to be higher than non-civil service scales, especially at the lower skill levels.

[20] Theodore W. Schultz, "Investment in Poor People," Seminar on Manpower Policy and Progress (Washington, Dept. of Labor, February 1967), p. 8.

Average wages for hospital personnel are also likely to be higher in areas with populations of one million or more, than in smaller communities. This relationship also holds when hospital size is taken into account. For example, the average weekly earnings for women general duty nurses in nonmetropolitan areas are lower than earnings in large metropolitan areas, and are lower too in smaller hospitals than in larger hospitals in nonmetropolitan areas.[21]

We wish to point out, however, that on the basis of data developed in our own survey, to which we have already referred, we did not find any pronounced tendency of wages to vary with hospital size (measured by bed complement). We examined data which are based on a more detailed size breakdown than the less-than or more-than 500-employee criterion used by the BLS in its 1966 survey, in order to determine with greater precision, the relationship of wage rate to hospital size. Our review of the data suggests that type of control and supply–demand relationships weigh much more heavily than size of hospital, among the several causal factors involved in wage differentials.

The foregoing analysis of wage levels and changes was based on average straight-time weekly or hourly earnings. No attention has been paid to fringe benefits, shift differentials, perquisites, and the like. In the short run, where wage rates are approximately equal, these factors may be determining so far as interregional or intra-regional mobility is concerned. Over time, however, one would expect that regional competition would affect the other items in the same way as it does basic wage rates.

Since specialization is continuing and new health occupations are appearing as a consequence, it is important to include them in any comprehensive analysis. To date, many of the newer occupations are not included in the BLS averages from which much of the

---

[21] "Earnings of Hospital Nurses, July, 1966," *Monthly Labor Review*, Vol. 90, No. 6 (June 1967), p. 55.

foregoing data are derived. Table 5.6 presents some of these occupations together with representative salaries so that the reader may obtain some notion of where they fit in the allied health wage structure.

Table 5.6

Representative Salaries of Newer Allied Health Occupations

Median Weekly Salary	Occupation	Area	Date
$130.20	Radio isotope technician	New York City	1967
129.69	Nurse anesthetist	Arizona	1965
115.61	Chief inhalation therapist (registered)	Delaware Valley	1967
103.15	Operating room surgical nurse	Los Angeles	1965
84.69	Operating room nurse	Arizona	1965
80.76	Electro-encephalograph technician	Denver	1965
80.76	Operating room surgical technician	Los Angeles	1965
80.76	Tissue technician	Denver	1965
78.00	Staff inhalation therapist (nonregistered)	Delaware Valley	1967
77.30	Electro-cardiograph technician	Los Angeles	1965
56.76	Dark-room technician	Denver	1965
52.78	Pharmacy helper	Denver	1965

To the above list should be added such health occupations as, dental laboratory technicians, environmental health specialists, rehabilitation therapists, orthoptists, and the like.

Unemployment Rates of Allied Health Personnel

A labor market analysis would be incomplete without some attention having been paid to the question of unemployment. For information of this kind we must revert to census data, since unemployment rates on a detailed medical occupational level and on a current basis are nonexistent.

Accordingly, we calculated unemployment rates for a variety of health occupations by subtracting those employed from the experienced civilian labor force and dividing that number by the experienced civilian labor force once again. This procedure was done for both 1950 and 1960.

The general view we obtained from these data is that, on the whole, unemployment rates in the medical occupations are much lower than they are in the economy at large. Indeed, zero rates and rates below one percent appear with great frequency, indicating a situation of virtual overemployment—one in which there is not enough flexibility to allow for job changing. Finally, it should be observed that it is only in the occupations requiring little training that relatively high unemployment rates were frequently seen.

The notion of a shortage or of overemployment is supported by recent pilot studies of job vacancies. Not only do occupations such as registered nurse, laboratory technician, physical therapist, and licensed practical nurse show high vacancy rates, but they are of the "hard-to-fill" type, that is to say, they are vacancies which remained unfilled for at least a month.[22]

Additional supportive evidence of shortages of allied health manpower is provided by the results of the Public Health Service– American Hospital Association survey of hospital staffing needs, completed in 1966. There were "urgent unmet needs" in hospital manpower (exclusive of physicians) for a 30 percent increase in occupational therapy workers, a 16 percent increase in professional nurses, a 15 percent increase in physical therapists and a 12 percent increase in licensed practical nurses.[23]

[22] National Bureau of Economic Research, *The Measurement and Interpretation of Job Vacancies* (New York, Columbia University Press, 1966), pp. 55 and 391.

[23] Neal H. Rosenthal, "The Health Manpower Gap: A High Hurdle," in *Occupational Outlook Quarterly,* Vol. 11, No. 1 (February 1967), p. 2.

Labor Market Efficiency

In the area of medical employment, the difficulty of matching workers and jobs is compounded by the occupational stratification, often backed by law, which is characteristic of this field. As indicated, a tight labor market brought about by the greatly expanded (and expanding) demand for health services, meliorates this situation to some extent, but there are distinct limits to the market's effectiveness. Additional leverage is needed at the legislative level as well as at the level of organizational change to loosen up the rigidly (and often anachronistically) defined job demarcations without, of course, incurring a quality trade-off.

In the short run, labor market problems center around the techniques for disseminating information on job vacancies for "qualified" personnel, on attempts to upgrade workers whose on-the-job experience qualifies them for better positions, and on recruiting inexperienced and untrained workers for the many entry level health jobs as aides, assistant helpers, and maintenance workers.

Technically trained workers (X-ray, laboratory, etc.) experience little difficulty currently in obtaining employment not only because of the supply–demand imbalance but because of informational sources available to them, informally by their co-workers and more formally by their association publications. (This is one of the positive aspects of the professionalization drive.)

As far as other communication channels are concerned, the tight labor market, which tends to reduce or to eliminate entirely the requirement that the worker pay a fee for securing a job, has militated in favor of public employment agencies such as U.S. Employment Service and direct advertising by the employer (hospital, usually) in newspaper classified sections, over the private employment agencies and "registries." The specialized agency, which supplies part-time or temporary health workers, continues to show viability, however.

Barriers to interregional mobility still exist and are reinforced by the lack of reciprocity arrangements among states so far as licensure is concerned. Ostensibly, these barriers are designed to protect the public, but in many cases, they are merely devices which relatively high-wage areas use to insulate themselves from the incursions of personnel from low-wage areas. In a situation of rather general shortages, these practices require careful reexamination.

Part of the problem of improving and maintaining the efficiency with which labor markets operate is the provision for orderly collective bargaining procedures. Since unionization is on the threshold and since the professional organizations are becoming more militant in the economic area, new attitudes and constructive approaches to these problems by all parties are warranted—especially since the interests of the public are so vitally involved.

Conclusions

In many ways, as we have attempted to demonstrate, the medical labor market has adjusted by classic means to the relatively tight supply–demand situation since 1950. We have also pointed out areas where the expected adjustments have failed to take place or have done so with considerable stickiness. For a number of reasons on the demand side, it is our view that the needs (effective demands) for medical and especially for allied health personnel will continue to grow rapidly, and although wages will also continue to rise, whether they will do so in the next few years at the same rates as they have in the recent past, is a matter of conjecture.

The major problems on the supply side are, first, the need to expand the medical labor force now through efforts to induce experienced workers to return to work and, second, to train new workers for health jobs. An evaluation of some of the attempts to accomplish these objectives is presented in Chapter 7.

Finally, we cannot limit our concern to the quantity factor; the quality dimension is equally important. But quality depends not only on the training and capacities of the individual worker, but on how he is utilized with other workers and with physical inputs to produce the health care product. In short, we must be concerned with overall efficiency. The relative insularity of the hospital from market pressures—pressures which often result in improved efficiency—is breaking down. What we need, as Schultz points out, are "ideas to identify and correct, now that we have a strong labor market, all manner of misuses of labor that are a part of the price of yesterday's slack and of our unpreparedness for today's aggregate demand." [24]

[24] Schultz, p. 7.

CHAPTER 6

Facets of Utilization

THIS STUDY is concerned mainly with understanding the forces leading to an increase in the supply of allied health workers in health institutions. However neither the supply and training of these workers, nor the behavior of the health labor market, can be fully understood without some reference to the existing manner of utilization of allied health personnel. The structure of the industry forms a general framework which is sometimes advantageous and sometimes disadvantageous to the development of allied health occupations.

The general outline of the health services industry has been sketched in earlier chapters. A brief recapitulation would be useful here.

Medical services must be supplied at the local level throughout the country. The geographical scattering of health institutions poses problems relating to the distribution and geographical mobility of health service workers. In addition, a wide variety of skills is needed in each location. Increasingly, each skill is invested in a different individual, giving rise to a large number of separate occupations, each organized, however loosely, on a professional model. Wherever there are professional or quasi-professional occupations, each distinct but working in close conjunction with the others, there is inevitable slippage in the efficient utilization of all due to assertions of professional hegemony and resultant interprofessional rivalry.

The historical origins of health care institutions are not to be found in the profit-making or business sector of the economy; indeed, they were barely within the money economy at all. Funds were received not as payments but as charitable donations; work was performed not for wages but as a religious obligation or a voluntary service. Although patients now pay and workers are paid, the eleemosynary syndrome persists. Construction is frequently financed by philanthropic donations, and large-scale operating deficits are not unusual. During 1966, for example, in-service volunteer workers contributed 2,456,599 hours of service to 78 voluntary and municipal hospitals in New York City. In the 62 member-hospitals of the United Hospital Fund, income from contributions amounted to 3.6 percent of the operating budget. Two hospitals reported deficits of over a million dollars. This traditional dependence on philanthropy has adversely affected attitudes toward capital and manpower and toward the utilization of the human resources of the industry. Efficiency of operation has not been a priority concern. Despite public demands for economy, hospitals are ultimately judged by the quantity and quality of the services they provide, not by the efficiency with which they are provided. And the call for more services is louder than the call for lower costs.

The large proportion of women workers in health services adds to the complexity of the utilization problem, particularly with reference to length of service and career development.

Problems of Utilization

Hospitals and health services employment have been expanding rapidly for some time and will continue to expand. Although in aggregate terms one can talk about a 54 percent increase between 1950 and 1960 (see Chapter 2), in terms of the individual hospital one must look at it as one new job in the X-ray department, two new places in the lab, three more people in nursing services, etc. Increments in employment usually take place one or two at a time, as the gradually increased demand for services causes a gradually increased need for workers.

Just as expansion in the individual institution takes place incrementally, so also do shortages develop slowly, and steps to deal with them are taken one at a time. As the departments struggle to increase services and the hospital board struggles to keep down costs, the cry is heard: "Just one more assistant, just one more aide, just one more technician is all we need to get things done." Only a sudden and massive increase in needs, such as the opening of a new hospital, a new wing, or a new service is likely to lead to a rational calculation of total manpower needs and an attempt to reorganize services.

Many of the new services and institutions being developed are a less expensive alternative to costly hospital care. Nursing homes and outpatient clinics, for example, which require fewer employees per patient, are increasing in number. However, as each of these facilities expands, it too faces the problem of "just one more assistant."

Each institution must attempt to meet the shortage of manpower as it arises. Demands for more training facilities do not produce new workers at the gates, and the hospitals have to accommodate to what is possible.

Manpower shortages exist, on the whole, among the more highly trained personnel. Unskilled workers are not in short supply. As any industry does, hospitals make use of the personnel available. The increased use of lower-level personnel has been well documented.[1]

Not all the work of a hospital, however, can be performed by un-

[1] Jeffrey Weiss, "The Changing Structure of Health Manpower" (unpublished dissertation, Harvard University, 1966).

skilled personnel. If a hospital cannot find enough trained personnel, it will often train its own. It frequently must do so since the
skills needed are not those that can be pirated from another industry. The training given will usually be specific to the needs of the
training institution and not easily transferable to another institution
(see Chapter 4). But hospitals are basically health service institutions and not schools, and despite ubiquitous training programs,
highly trained workers are still in short supply.

One response to the shortage of personnel is the hiring of part-
time personnel. Nationally, about 14 percent of hospital personnel
were part time in 1964. Fincher estimated that over half of the hospitals in Georgia used part-time medical technologists. It has been
estimated that 20 percent of the dental assistants and 55 percent of
the dental hygienists are on part-time schedules. A survey in Wisconsin showed from 13 to 28 percent of the technician and "assistant" occupations were filled with part-time workers.[2]

Part-time work is especially prevalent among nursing personnel,
as the data in Table 6.1 reveal. It would appear that part-time employment is more prevalent among the higher than among the
lower-skilled personnel, and more prevalent in smaller institutions.
Smaller hospitals, for example, are less likely to have a trained dietician, and if they do, she is more likely to be a part-time worker.

It was shown in one study that only 3.7 percent of hospitals with
a bed complement of 25 or less employed a full-time dietician,
whereas in the 300 to 400 bed range, over 77 percent of the hospitals did so.[3] It is not uncommon for a trained worker to split her

[2] *Hospitals: Journal of the American Hospital Association,* Vol. 39, Part 2,
Guide Issue (August 1965); Cameron Fincher, *Nursing and Paramedical Personnel in Georgia* (Atlanta, Georgia State College, 1962); "Job Development
and Training for Workers in Health Services," *Background Data Book* (Washington, Dept. of Labor and Dept. of Health, Education, and Welfare, 1966), pp.
102–4; *A Study of Health and Related Service Occupations in Wisconsin* (Madi-
son, Wisconsin State Employment Service, 1964).

[3] "Food Service Management in Hospitals," *Journal of the American Dietician's
Association* (April 1965), p. 256.

time between two institutions which can pay for her services only on a part-time basis.

But part-time work in large institutions is also common as a response to shortage of personnel. It would be difficult to judge the extent to which part-time workers could be used in the various departments. A certain proportion of workers must be full time for continuity of administration. Hospitals have functioned, albeit with difficulties, with up to 75 percent of the nursing staff on part time.

Table 6.1

Part-Time Nursing Personnel
As Percent of Total Nursing Personnel, 1966

	Professional Nurses	Licensed Practical Nurses	Nurse's Aides
Short-term general hospital	26	11	no data
Osteopathic hospital	30	9	12
Nursing homes	25	21	14

Source: *Facts About Nursing, 1966.*

Hospitals on the whole are reluctant to use part-time workers because of the interruption of the routine, the discontinuity of responsibility, and the high cost of administration. As was indicated in the previous chapter, only 18 percent of the workers in "medical and other health services" in the nation in 1965 were part-time workers. This may be contrasted with 32 percent in welfare and religious, 22 percent in educational services, and 34 percent in retail trade. It is, of course, much higher than in manufacturing (5 percent). In times of shortage, however, the part-time workers are better than no workers. A revision of schedule, so that mothers can work when their children are in school or provision made for children to be cared for at the work site, would enable more employers to take advantage of these labor resources.

Problems of Turnover

Beyond the actual shortage of manpower lies the shortage created by high turnover, causing many jobs to be vacant for varying periods of time. High turnover of personnel has been a feature of health service employment for a long time. Nevertheless, surprisingly little data on turnover has been collected.

Turnover is usually measured as the number of separations during a year divided by the number of workers at the beginning of the year; e.g., if there are 30 workers at the beginning and 15 quit during the year, the turnover rate is 50 percent.

A national survey by the Catholic Hospital Association in 1958 of industrial areas found an average turnover of 83 percent. An estimate of New York City voluntary hospitals in 1959 found turnover varying from 34 to 90 percent among the hospitals. A national survey of psychiatric aides showed an average turnover of 30 percent, with the higher turnover in the smaller institutions.[4] A Georgia survey of turnover among professional personnel found a variation of from 9 to 38 percent in the various health occupations. A large New York City hospital noted for the stability of its work force shows an annual turnover of from 20 to 39 percent among allied health personnel. (The implementaion of recommendations of a management consultant firm was largely responsible for this relatively low rate.)

Turnover rates are somewhat deceptive and should be measured against stability, or the numbers of workers present at the beginning of the year who were still there at the end. A detailed examination of the turnover in a large general New York City hospital shows this relationship (Table 6.2). In the nursing department, 166 out of the 218 jobs were filled by the same people throughout the year, producing a stability rate of 76 percent. The remaining 52

---

[4] *Hospital Personnel* (Washington, Public Health Service, 1964); *The Psychiatric Aide in State Mental Hospitals* (Washington, Public Health Service, 1965).

Table 6.2

Turnover and Stability in a New York Hospital

	1 Work Force at Beginning of Year	2 Stable Work Force	3 Stability Rate (1 ÷ 2)	4 Unstable Work Force	5 No. of Turnovers	6 General Turnover Rate (5 ÷ 1)	7 Turnover Rate in Unstable Jobs * (5 ÷ 4)
Department							
Nursing	218	166	76%	52	107	49%	206%
Auxiliary nursing	290	234	81	56	88	30	157
Social service	26	22	85	4	10	39	250
Laboratory	72	49	68	23	27	38	117
Medical Records	27	22	81	5	11	33	220
Physical medicine	16	13	81	3	7	44	233
Radiology	58	42	72	16	16	28	100

* 100% = each job turned over only once.

jobs were filled and emptied several times, bringing the turnover rate, which is measured in people, not jobs, to 46 percent.

We were not able to obtain historical information for this hos‧ pital, which would give the data previous to the intervention of the hospital consultant. However, another New York City hospital, St. Vincent's, published a report of its experience with management consultants which showed that with good management, not only turnover, but low morale and costly inefficiency can be reduced. The hospital traced a large part of its excessive turnover to poor job structure, overlapping and discontinuous authority, poor wage policy, insufficient job training, and the like. The changes that were introduced brought St. Vincent's turnover rate down from 74 percent in 1956 to 26 percent in 1963, where it has remained. The turnover rates in the nursing and other health departments for 1958, 1959 (when the program was completed), and 1966 are particularly noteworthy (Table 6.3).

Table 6.3

Turnover Rates at St. Vincent's Hospital

	1958	1959	1966
Laboratory	44.7	44.2	34.1
Medical records	78.3	40.4	42.2
Nutrition	77.1	35.5	35.5
Radiology	73.2	38.0	41.2
Social service	23.6	20.9	22.9
Mental health	29.0	9.7	21.9
Nursing	65.5	54.2	37.6
Nurse's aides			32.6
Nursing technicians			23.1
RN and LPN			44.9

Source: *Hospital Personnel* (Washington, Public Health Service, 1964).

Although the cost of the program was high, the cost of turnover is also high. St. Vincent's estimated that the reduction in turnover between 1958 and 1959 alone produced a direct saving to the hospital of $45,000.

Several facts become clear from the listing of turnover in these two hospitals. First, that the highest turnover rates are among registered nurses, in comparison with whom the auxiliary nursing and other health personnel are fairly stable. Second, the turnover in hospitals will remain relatively high no matter what steps are taken, due to the nature of the work force. It has been estimated that there is a "hard core" of unavoidable turnover of 20 to 25 percent in hospitals which is due to factors outside the work system, such as family or health problems. The large number of women accounts for much of the turnover due to family obligations. Unfortunately we could not unearth turnover statistics broken down by age, sex, and marital status, but most indicators seem to point to the concentration of young, single females as responsible for much of the mobility.[5] The high turnover rate is also a function of the small size of the establishments, their geographical dispersion, and the specificity of occupation. These factors will be covered more fully later in the chapter.

The third point that emerges is that turnover can be reduced to a workable minimum through a rationalization of the job structure. For one thing, many hospitals do not keep turnover statistics and are unaware of its extent. For another, most hospitals are not aware of the hidden costs of turnover in terms of work lost, supervising and other time spent in training, and the burden placed on other workers to keep things running until the replacement arrives.

The extent of the impact that employee turnover can have on hospital costs is illustrated by the following conclusion of a recent study by the United Hospital Fund of New York: "The minimum direct cost of replacing a competent worker probably ranges from

[5] Phil Smith, "The Influence of Wage Rates on Nurse Mobility" (University of Chicago, Graduate School of Business, Institute of Industrial and Labor Relations).

300 to 700 times the hourly pay cost for that position. . . . Direct costs, considerable as they are, when we multiply them by the 36 percent to 72 percent of the numbers of the payroll who separate annually, are small compared with the indirect costs of avoidable turnover and resulting understaffing." [6]

Another reason for the lack of concern is that high turnover has been present for as long as shortages have, and the hospitals have come to accept it as unchangeable. In some cases it is seen as an alternative to high wages, and therefore preferable.

The institutions which tend to be in the forefront of research in all areas also tend to be those which are well run and pay high wages, and therefore less likely to have a shortage of workers or to have excessive turnover of staff. They do not feel as much need for research on turnover as do the less well-situated hospitals, and the latter often cannot afford the investment in research that a solution would require.

Shortages and excessive turnover are not the cause of problems as much as they are the result of long standing factors in the health service industry. One of the most obvious—wages—has been covered in the previous chapter. Less obvious, but of major importance, are several other factors which will be covered in the remainder of the chapter. They are organizational structure of health service institutions, the professionalism of health occupations, and the career mobility of health workers.

Administrative Structure

The most influential working group in hospitals and health services is the physicians. So long as they have superior technical competence and the ultimate responsibility for the patients, they will continue to have predominant power in health organizations. This situ-

---

[6] United Hospital Fund of New York, "Analyzing and Reducing Employee Turnover in Hospitals," *Study Report #3* (New York, 1968), p. 6.

ation tends to weaken the role of administrators. Nurses supervise nurses, physicians supervise physicians, chief technicians supervise other technicians, and higher ranking professions supervise lower ranking professions. Furthermore, as one sociologist put it, "The existence of many exceptions . . . increases both the power and the discretion of the technical group which handles these exceptions, at the expense of the supervisory group." [7] By "exceptions" the author means cases that cannot easily be routinized. In organizational terms, the "staff is not separated from the "line"; it is the "line."

Such arrangements may produce the most direct service to the patients, but create havoc with the organizational structure. Professionals, by their nature, are unconcerned with administration, and as hospitals grow larger, the problems of uncoordination, duplicated authority, and tangled lines of communication also grow larger. The importance of good management for the delivery of health services has been underestimated.

An increasing rationalization of structure is taking place, and several new occupations have arisen to deal with it. In this connection, mention should be made of the increasing importance of unit clerks, ward supervisors, administrative assistants, and hospital administrators, the last named trained for their jobs in graduate schools. Increasing awareness of the administration problem is shown by the increase of these occupations as well as in the increasing use made by hospitals of management consulting firms.

Except for the hospital administrators, who are increasingly important to the management of hospitals, the new occupations deal mainly with routine clerical tasks that the professionals slough off. For the vast majority of medical and allied health workers, supervision and authority will continue to be distributed by technical rank, and the hierarchy of professions will constitute the hierarchy of rank and power.

[7] Charles Perrow, "A Framework for the Comparative Analyses of Organizations," *American Sociological Review*, Vol. 32, No. 2 (April, 1967), p. 200.

This has many obvious advantages, but also has some equally relevant disadvantages. The process of professionalization has produced a large number of separate occupations with fairly impermeable barriers between them. This has decreased the possibilities of upward mobility to a point at which it has become a serious problem (see Chapter 5).

Vertical Mobility

The concept of upward mobility, and its blockage, due to professionalism, should be examined in detail. Upward mobility can be loosely defined as rising in income, prestige, acknowledged responsibilities, and skills.

Where self-employment is common, one "rises" only to the extent of establishing a successful business or practice and earning more income and prestige. Doctors, dentists, pharmacists, optometrists, and psychologists frequently follow this route. In the occupations in which one is employed by an institution, there are several forms of mobility. The first, the professional model, is similar to the self-employed model. One remains in the occupation as a practitioner and rises in rank or in prestige within the institution. Hospital administrators, biochemists, dieticians are examples here. This is the "ideal" model for the employed professional, one that is followed alike by academicians and medical researchers.

There are basically two other routes for employed workers. The first is to rise in administrative responsibility, either within the occupation or above the occupation. This is the route taken by professional nurses, who, because they are responsible for much of the day-to-day administration in the hospital, have a clearly defined administrative hierarchy up to, and sometimes including, the hospital administrator. Social workers are also able to move up into the administration of departments or agencies, although their greatest opportunities are not within the hospitals. This, of course, is only possible when there is an administrative hierarchy through which to climb. The second route is to shift or change occupations to one on a higher level. A nurse might become a nurse-anesthetist; an orderly, an EEG technician; a laboratory technologist, a nuclear medical technologist.

There are, then, four main possibilities. For the "independent" professional, mobility comes through increased incomes and prestige within the occupation; if self-employed, through building a successful practice, if employed, through increased rank and prestige of the institution. For the nonindependent or salaried worker, one who by definition works under someone else in a hierarchical arrangement, mobility comes either through rising in the administrative structure or through rising to a higher level occupation, either vertically or diagonally.

The vast majority of allied health workers are employed by institutions. They cannot rise in the administrative structure because there is none separate from the professional structure. It is virtually impossible to rise to a higher occupational level because of the very long training periods involved. For example, a physical therapy assistant who wished to become a physical therapist would have to spend four years in full-time education. A therapist or technician in a large institution could rise one level to chief therapist or chief technician, but above that level, there is a different profession—the physiologist, radiologist, or pathologist. Among the lower-level occupations there is not even a chief, supervision being performed directly by a member of a higher-ranking occupation.

Even mobility in terms of pay raises and grade levels is limited by the small number of workers in each occupation employed in each establishment. Table 6.4 demonstrates the lack of promotion possibilities within allied health occupations. Less than 50 percent of the workers in each occupation are working in an occupational structure which permits promotion. The low proportion of workers holding supervisory posts is also notable.

Table 6.4

Promotion Possibilities for Selected Allied Health Personnel

	No Promotion Possible (Single grade only)	Promotion Possible		Supervisory Grades	Not Reported
		Nonsupervisory Grades			
		lowest	middle and higher		
Laboratory technicians, specified	50.5	18.2	25.6	5.6	
Laboratory technicians, general	51.1	18.2	18.6	4.4	7.5
X-ray and related technicians	55.8	20.2	17.0	6.7	.3
Therapists	56.8	17.4	17.8	8.0	
Medical records librarians	62.2	13.8	8.1	15.9	
Other technicians (EKG, inhalation, therapist, etc.)	78.8	8.4	9.2	2.5	
Dental laboratory technicians	77.0	4.4	14.6	3.7	.3
Dental hygienists	98.3	.6	1.0	.1	
Dental assistants	97.5	.4	2.0	.04	
Medical assistants	100.0				

Source: "Technical Manpower in New York State," *Special Bulletin 239* (N.Y. State Dept. of Labor, December 1964), Vol I, Supp. A, Table 17.

Some upward mobility is possible. Unskilled workers can move upward to the semi-skilled or low technical levels as the training time is not prohibitive. The majority of operating room technicians, inhalation therapists, EKG and EEG technicians are orderlies or nurse's aides who have been trained on the job. A recent survey of dental hygienists found that 16 percent had previously been dental assistants.[8]

A few steps are being taken to increase mobility, but they have not, on the whole, been very effective. MDTA largely prepares people for entry into jobs in unskilled, semi-skilled and low level technical work and provides some upward mobility for the already employed. The "New Careers" program for the indigenous nonprofessional attempts to build career ladders from low- to high-skilled work, but the administrators are finding that organizations are more frequently willing to provide the lower-level job than the mobility ladder. Some union agreements insist on promotion ladders for the union members into jobs of medium skill.[9]

A few hospitals are providing ladders for their employees, but they only go from the lowest rung to the next lowest rung. The stumbling block in all of these is the high educational requirement for each occupation and the lack of transferability of training.

A person trained in one health specialty cannot transfer his skills to a related specialty on the same level, but must go back to the beginning and retake the entire training program. At present, the most usual means of improving one's position is to change to higher-paying jobs at the same level in a different institution. An important factor is the dispersal of work units, making it frequently necessary to change geographical location in order to change jobs. A study of census data on all professional, technical, and kindred workers

[8] Robert G. Kessel and M. Holmquist, "Survey of Dentistry: Report on Dental Hygienists," *Journal of the American Dental Hygienists Association* (January 1961), pp. 9–21.

[9] See, for example, the recent contract between New York City and the American Federation of State, County, and Municipal Employers, November, 1966.

found that "for numerous salaried professionals a combination of highly marketable skills, blunted organizational advancement, and decentralized work units fosters high rates of migration." [10]

Another common means of upward mobility is leaving the occupation altogether. In 1954, the American Registry of X-Ray Technicians surveyed the 2,739 registered technicians no longer working in the X-ray field: 1,620 were housewives; the remaining 919 were distributed as shown in Table 6.5.

Table 6.5

Occupational Distribution of
Former X-ray Technicians

	Number	*Percent*
Salesmen, including X-ray	116	12.6
Office workers, nonmedical	160	17.4
Engineers	56	6.1
Physicians or medical students	40	4.3
Hospital administrators	62	6.8
Professional nurses	22	2.4
Dentists, pharmacists	15	1.6
Anesthetists	14	1.5
Other health personnel (20 fields)	61	6.6
Elementary school teachers	17	1.9
College teachers	47	4.0
Agricultural workers	24	2.6
Personnel, nonmedical	9	1.0
Priests, ministers, missionaries	8	0.9
Self-employed (38 fields)	53	5.8
Misc. employment (22 fields)	39	4.2
Students	89	9.7
Retired	26	2.8
Unemployed	71	7.7

Source: Alfred Green, "Quo Fata Vacant," *X-ray Technicians,* XXVI (September 1954), 87.

[10] Jack Ladinsky, "Occupational Determinants of Geographic Mobility Among Professional Workers," *American Sociological Review,* Vol. 32 (April, 1967).

In 1954, when this survey was taken, many of the previous members had been licensed by examination only, with skills learned on the job. Since there were few formal educational requirements, workers could use it as a steppingstone, a part-time or night job while attending college. Even today, many X-ray technicians trained by the Army follow this route upon separation. But as formal requirements rise, this route is closed. Few people will attend two years of X-ray school to put themselves through college afterwards.

Some changes are now taking place in the structure of health services which may lead to increased mobility within the field. Mobility to high-level occupations is and will remain difficult due to expense, although scholarship aid and training funds will alleviate this somewhat. But mobility through administrative channels is becoming increasingly possible. The trend toward contracting-out certain services opens opportunities in the administrative structure of the external service companies.[11] There is also increasing opportunity for allied health workers as administrators in nursing homes and clinics, which on the whole are not large enough to require the full-time administration of a physician. As hospitals grow in size, the previously mentioned increase in clerical and administrative personnel may open opportunities at all levels. In one experiment, the University of Michigan hospital has separated completely the administrative staff and the nursing staff, making parallel structures. Such an arrangement provides two mobility routes; one professional, the other administrative. Nurse's aides, practical nurses, and other allied health workers may be enabled to transfer into the administrative staff and to rise within it.

[11] Harry I. Greenfield, *Manpower and the Growth of Producers Services* (New York, Columbia University Press, 1966.

The Role of Professionalism

The importance of professions in health services cannot be under-rated. No other industry contains such a large number of different types of professions at such different levels of skills. Whether the majority of occupations constitute "true" professions in the socio-logical sense is unimportant here; the importance lies in the use of the professional model by the members of the occupation and in the effect on the industry of the use of this model.

The justification for professionalism is that the worker has unique competence to deal with a given process, structure, or situa-tion which is important to the community but potentially danger-ous in the hands of an incompetent. Because of the supposed unique competence involved, control over the profession should be in the hands of the professionals. The three most important aspects of control are *training* the new members; *certifying* the competence of those allowed to practice; and *regulating* the quality of practice of the members. Thus the various professional organizations of physicians, including the AMA, control the training of new physi-cians through accreditation of medical schools, control the certifica-tion of newcomers through state laws, specialty boards, and the like, and regulate the quality of practice through official committees on medical ethics and malpractice and through approval of hospitals for internships and residencies.[12]

Many allied health professions have modeled themselves after the physicians and other high-level independent professions. They have tried to accredit only the schools meeting their minimum qualifications and to prevent nonaccredited schools from function-ing. They have set minimum certification requirements for begin-ning workers and have attempted to prevent uncertified people

[12] See "Medical Education in the United States, 1966–67," *Journal of the Amer-ican Medical Association,* Vol. 202, No. 8 (November 20, 1967).

from working either through the voluntary acquiescence of their employers or through state laws. They have promulgated codes of ethics and asserted their right to bar miscreants from practice. These attempts have met with varying degrees of success. At least 20 allied health occupations have some accredited training programs. The existence of unaccredited programs is difficult to uncover. A better indicator of the extent of success is the proportion of workers who are certified by a professional society or legal body, since such certification usually, though not always, requires graduation from an accredited school. Estimates here are also difficult to make. Data gathered from *Health Resources Statistics 1965* show the approximate distribution of certification for those allied health workers for whom data was available.

Workers	Percent Certified
Occupational therapists	86
Physical therapists	67
Orthotics and Prosthetics makers	33
X-ray technicians	40
Medical social workers	50
Psychiatric social workers	75
Medical librarians	9
Medical records librarians	12
Dental hygienists	100
Dental assistants	4
Dental technicians	24
Clinical laboratory technicians	43
Dieticians and nutritionists	40
Inhalation therapists	5
Electroencephalograph technicians	1

These figures can be misleading. For example, although only 9 percent of the medical librarians are certified, over 35 percent have professional library training. In medical technology, 43 percent are registered but an additional 5 percent have higher educational qualifications than are needed for registration.[13] Those occupations in which the percent certified is low have only recently formed certifying bodies. On the whole, the professionalizing movement is fairly recent, and many of the older members of the occupation were certified through so-called grandfather clauses. Thus Fincher found that among the licensed practical nurses in Georgia in 1962, a possible maximum of 63 percent had actually undergone the required one year's training (licensing began in 1953).

A recent survey of dental hygienists (Kessel and Holmquist) shows the influence of rising educational standards in the field. The present requirements for dental hygienists include two years of training, but this level has been reached slowly from the beginning in on-the-job training. The survey data showed that of those who have been working for thirty years or more, and thus are at least thirty years away from their original training, almost 90 percent had one year or less of training. And of the most recent graduates, 100 percent had the now-required two years. In between, the percentage with two years of training slowly increases from the early to the later years, so that at the time of the survey, over 60 percent of the dental hygienists had at least the required two years.

The analogous percentages in all occupations nationally have not been determined. Another difficulty is that these occupations frequently contain several levels of personnel, and only the highest level requires certification. To use a clear example from the nursing situation, 100 percent of the registered nurses are certified nurses, but they only constitute 44 percent of the employed nursing personnel. The inclusion of licensed practical nurses brings the certified portion to 64 percent.[14]

The ability of any professional organization to control the practice of its members, once certified, is low. No data are available in this area. However, professions can help to determine who will

[13] *Health Resources Statistics, 1965* (Washington, Public Health Service).
[14] *Facts About Nursing* (New York, American Nurses Association, 1966).

practice through the promulgation of state licensing laws. These may either restrict work in the occupation to those persons who have fulfilled the professional requirements, or they may just restrict the use of the professional title to certified graduates.

Licensing laws are quite difficult to enforce. If the work must be done, the hospitals will find a way of doing it—by assigning a non-professional to a professional position, by keeping him in a nonprofessional position but assigning the professional tasks to him, or by assigning titular "responsibility" to an absent physician. If a law were sufficiently watertight to detail exactly what acts could or could not be undertaken by specific people, it would also limit the ability of the institution to deliver services. In a situation of scarcity with a fast-changing occupational structure, limits on flexibility of personnel inhibit the development of more modern and efficient systems.

There are many reasons for the varying success of professionalization among allied health occupations, but most are an outgrowth of one main cause—the position of allied health workers in the professional hierarchy. The vast majority, as we have noted, are not independent but work under the supervision of the more highly educated members of a higher-ranking profession. It is difficult to claim unique competence when there exists in the field another professional body whose members have four, six, eight, or even ten years more education and training in the subject. Training is often performed by members of the higher-ranking profession; certification of lower-level workers is frequently in the hands of the higher-level professional society, and regulation of workers is accomplished through hiring, firing, and job recommendations of the higher-ranking professionals. The attitude of the higher-ranking profession is extremely important. If the higher-ranking profession puts its strength behind the lower-level society, achievement of professionalization is rapid, as was the case with dental hygienists. If the higher-ranking profession opposes the lower level's efforts, achievement is slowed considerably. There are sometimes three levels of personnel. In these cases the lowest level is sometimes in the same position vis-a-vis the middle level as the middle level is vis-a-vis the highest level; at other times the lowest level is directly related to the highest.

The widespread application of the professional model to the independent and dependent occupations in the health field is partially beneficial and partially detrimental to overall manpower utilization.

On the positive side, the professional societies' main efforts are devoted to raising the quality of workers in the field. The institution of accredited training programs assures that there will be training programs. It is not unusual for the superior professions to underestimate the skills needed in their subordinates, nor is it unusual for an institution to provide its trainees only with the skills needed in that institution. Professionally accredited training programs serve not only to raise the beginning competence of the workers but also to provide a fairly standard set of skills, enabling the workers to move to other institutions in search of better jobs. The certification procedure assures that there will be a certain percentage of well-trained "professionals" in the field. A 1966 study, *The Clinical Laboratory Improvement Program,* by the New York City Department of Labor showed that those clinical laboratories with the highest percentage of college graduates and registered medical technologists on their staffs were most likely to perform the correct diagnoses in a variety of routine tests. Several studies of X-ray technicians in New York and California have shown less awareness of safety precautions among nonregistered personnel.[15] Georgopolous and Mann, in their study of community hospitals, found that "material facilities per se do not play as crucial a role as do social

---

[15] See, for example, *Survey of X-ray Facilities, Current X-ray Safety Practices, and Teaching in California's Dental Assisting and Medical Assisting Schools* (California State Dept. of Public Health, 1965).

and psychological facilities in the skill and competence of organizational members, insofar as patient care is concerned." [16] Indeed, it would be difficult to imagine that lesser-trained workers would be likely to give better care.

The certification procedure also eases the problem of the hospital administrators and department heads who are responsible for hiring. The certification procedure is a guarantee of quality, or "seal of approval" for an incoming worker. Without it, each employer would have to be competent to judge the educational background of each worker when there are, as noted in Chapter 4, more than 50 occupations and several thousand training facilities.

It is also hoped that the professional society will succeed in instilling in each worker a professional attitude and pride in his work that will motivate him to adhere to professional ethics and to strive to improve his competence. The existence of a common professional body provides him with a type of independence from his immediate employer or his client and an orientation to the profession as a whole.

Professional journals and yearly conventions keep him informed of the latest developments. Since he may be the only one, or one of only a few, in his occupation at his hospital, this communication network may be important in keeping the quality of his work high.

In Robert N. Wilson's analysis, the lack of administrative structure and the emphasis on technical competence and professionalism combine to make each worker's prestige depend on his ability to produce. "With the exception of the lowest categories of hospital work, orderlies and aides, the general principle is that prestige hinges on the extent to which an individual's work entails direct patient care; in contrast to many other types of large organizations, the hospital community ranks a certain kind of manual labor—the production job or the assembly line—above almost all sorts of

[16] Basil S. Georgopolous and Floyd C. Mann, *The Community General Hospital* (New York, Macmillan, 1962).

white collar jobs." [17] Because there is no clear system of authority, there is a premium on flexible behavior, and each profession competes with the others to provide better service. The lower-ranking professions, in particular, attempt to raise their prestige by proving that they are essential for patient care. Thus, professionalization in many instances promotes the existence of initiative and responsibility on the part of workers.

There are a number of drawbacks to professionalism, and these are usually emphasized at the expense of the advantages. The members of each profession feel, not unnaturally, that they are the best qualified to do the work in their field. Each occupation tries to separate itself as far as possible from other occupations. As mentioned in Chapter 4, training for each occupation is very specific, making it virtually impossible for a worker trained in one occupation to transfer his skills to another occupation. The presence of the accredited training program cuts off, or attempts to cut off, the flow of workers from other training sources which may be equally valid such as the Armed Forces, private trade schools, or nonmedical graduate schools.

This also has the effect of leaving the field open to people whose training was totally outside the medical sphere. Medical professionals are unwilling to admit that nonmedical training can produce expertise. Indeed the attempt by pathologists to prevent chemists and biochemists from opening clinical laboratories has resulted in a Justice Department suit against an association of pathologists for combination in restraint of trade.[18]

It is also in the nature of professions to be wary of encroachment from below. When there is more than one level in a field, the levels tend to be widely separate, making upward mobility between levels virtually impossible. In the laboratory field, four years of

---

[17] Robert N. Wilson, "The Social Structure of a General Hospital," *Annals of the American Academy of Political and Social Science,* 346 (March 1963), 67–76.
[18] *The ASMT News,* November 1965.

medical school separate the pathologists from the next highest level, the medical technologists with, at most, a B.A. And at least three years of college separate the medical technologists from the certified laboratory assistants with only a high-school diploma. Usually the price extracted by the higher group for approving the lower group's organization is the promise that the lower-level workers will not compete with them and will work only under the direction of a member of the higher profession, which puts the lower level at a disadvantage with respect to wages and upward mobility.

The professions are often accused of trying to limit quantity and raise wages at a time when workers are in short supply. It must be pointed out that as long as the employers are free to hire uncertified workers—which they are, in the absence of state laws—professionalization cannot be seen as an artificial limit on supply. However, there is a strong tendency for health departments, professional organizations, or interested health agencies to try to impose state licensing in order to force standards up. The recent history of New York State with its 1965 licensing law for X-ray technicians is instructive.[19] At the time the law went into effect, 12,000 to 14,000 persons other than "physicians and other practitioners of the healing arts" were taking X-rays. Only 2,000 were registered with the American Registry of Radiologic Technologists.

During the past two years, about 6,800 practitioners have been licensed by the state, 2,500 on the basis of ARRT certification, the remainder by examination. New Yorkers are now assured that all persons working as X-ray technicians have passed tests of competence. However, X-rays are often taken in private physicians' offices. Whereas before the law, the physician's office assistant took the X-rays, now the physician himself must take them, even though he may have no more, and possibly even less, training in the specific

[19] Granville Larrimore, "New York State's X-Ray Technology Program," National Conference on X-Ray Technician Training (Washington, Public Health Service, 1966).

techniques of X-ray than his assistant. Private vocational schools which previously provided a good portion of the training for X-ray technicians and for the assistants in the office were virtually eliminated from the field although this was not legally necessary. Expansion of accredited schools did not begin until after the licensing laws took effect, with the resultant shortage of workers and a strong upsurge of wages.

The shortage of technicians and the resultant wage increases are expected to ease off as the accredited schools begin producing a sufficient number of graduates.

Summary

Only as the problems of the organization and efficient utilization of interdependent health personnel are solved will the "health industry" approach the model and levels of efficiency of other large industries. From the slight evidence available, it would appear that the problems considered in this chapter—the lack of adminstrative structure, ad hoc efforts to deal with shortages, high turnover of personnel, low upward mobility, and excessive separation of professions—have not become more real in the past few years, but just more apparent.

As the visibility of the problems has increased, so have efforts to deal with them. Increasing importance is paid to research and demonstration projects, many funded by the Public Health Service and by the Hospital Research and Educational Trust to rationalize the administrative structure of hospitals and to increase efficient utilization of personnel. Increasing attention is also being paid to reducing the high turnover rates and increasing the opportunity for upward career mobility among hospital workers. There are murmurings about increasing interprofessional cooperation at the organizational level. The presence of interdisciplinary programs in medical and dental schools and in schools for allied health professions, in which workers in many different occupations are trained in close proximity, may help to increase interprofessional cooperation and understanding at the working level. Some consideration is being given to reducing the chaos of conflicting state regulations concerning health personnel.

These few steps are only the beginning, and it would be unrealistic to consider that the multitudinous problems in these areas will be solved in the near future. Some are due to the legacy of poor planning in the past; some are due to the inertia of the present; but many are an integral part of the nature of the industry and the needs of its consumers. The delivery of health services will continue to be scattered through a large number of locations throughout the country. As facilities become increasingly available, people will make increasing use of them, and there will in one sense always be a "shortage" with its concomitant problems.

A high priority must be placed on the effective utilization of existing personnel both to increase the amount of services of which the system is presently capable as well as serving as a model for the training and absorption of new workers.

CHAPTER 7

Federal Programs

IN THE 170 years or so since the establishment of the Public Health Service via a "bill for the relief of sick and disabled seamen," [1] federal activities affecting health have extended to virtually every department of government and, through intergovernmental activities, to every region in the nation. Our task here is not to review that long history nor even to discuss the rationale of government activity in health, rather it is to outline and evaluate those activities which, directly or indirectly, affect allied health personnel as distinct from the core group.

It is useful, for this purpose to treat the civilian and military aspects separately with the full appreciation that there are many points of overlap.

Military Programs

First, with respect to the military side of the picture, there are a number of important points to be made and lessons to be learned:

1. Almost by definition, the military establishment has a control over manpower disposition and utilization not possessed by any other segment of our society. With congressional authorization, it

[1] Harry S. Mustard, *Government in Public Health*, Studies of the New York Academy of Medicine, Committee on Medicine and the Changing Order (New York, The Commonwealth Fund, 1945), p. 26.

can recruit (conscript) men, train them, assign them, and reassign them—in short its control over its members is virtually absolute.

2. The military establishment is obligated to provide medical care to its members in the same way as it is obligated to provide food, clothing, and shelter. By the nature of its operations, whether during peace or war, the armed forces are not evenly distributed geographically, and many posts are established in remote areas with few personnel. Since there are not enough career physicians, dentists, and nurses to service all of these areas (or ships at sea as the case may be), the armed forces were forced to rely heavily on allied health personnel. Nor are the military constrained by all the various rules and regulations of the professional associations which operate in the civilian medical scene. It is therefore interesting to observe that under the pressures of need and of freedom from restraint, the military medical production function (see Chapter 1) exhibits a marked difference from its civilian counterpart, a difference which, for the most part, centers on a relatively greater utilization of allied health personnel. Further, since health personnel are not found in large numbers among draftees and enlistees, the military are again forced to provide their own supply through their own training devices. Here lies another important lesson. While military training manuals and instructors may not be models of pedagogical exposition, the end product is a health worker who can work effectively in the limited areas of his specialty. This comes about through a minute functional breakdown of medical operations and the performance of a task "by the numbers."

Of importance too is the fact that most military courses are of relatively short duration, and many are of the on-the-job training variety (see Table 7.1). This raises a host of questions that one may ask regarding the possibly undue length of training periods of various types of health personnel in the civilian sector. The fact is that in some of the occupations, such as X-ray technician, dental laboratory technician, and therapist, the civilian accrediting orga-

field is a formidable one. Apart from sex is the question of salary, and here again the wage levels in many health occupations are not generally conducive to recruitment of ex-military personnel. In addition, while the military almost invariably provides for upward mobility—through its system of grades, ranks, or classes—the civilian structure as we have seen, is notably devoid of such mechanisms. Another point here is the fact that there exist at present no precise civilian counterparts of certain military health occupations such as the medical corpsman. In many cases where the civilian counterpart does exist, the military health specialist is not automatically granted certification.

The military model is important then for three reasons: one is the vast utilization of allied health personnel in the production of health services (and this includes delivery systems as well); the second has to do with the potential for shortening course duration for civilian health occupations; and the third has to do with the potential for augmenting the supply of civilian health personnel through better articulation between the two systems.

Civilian Programs

The vast majority of civilian medical manpower programs have historically been associated with the U.S. Public Health Service. Generally, the demands on the Public Health Service are not of the same order of urgency as they are on the military, hence it does not undertake the same magnitude and kinds of training programs mentioned above. However, in terms of medical manpower utilization, the Public Health Service by virtue of the same chronic shortage of physicians was forced to rely increasingly on the Public Health Nurse to perform many of the services usually reserved for physicians and, in this way, contributed to a better understanding of the role of medical personnel with less than a physician's training. Some training of allied health manpower does take place in hospitals which are controlled by the Public Health Service in order to insure an adequate supply.

The first explicit attention paid to allied health personnel as a group by the federal government occurred in a section of the report "Building America's Health" in 1952.[2] That report devoted a separate section of its discussion of Health Personnel to "Paramedical Personnel." We might add parenthetically that there has not, since that time, been any thorough review of allied health personnel with the same depth as has been done subsequently in the case of physicians and nurses.[3]

A good overview of the federal government's involvement in medical manpower training is provided by an examination of the most recent Budget of the United States.[4] Health Expenditures are broken down into six functional categories: Grants and Payments for Medical Care, Direct Patient Care, Research, Training (including training for research), Preventive and Community Services, and Construction of Health Facilities.

Our focus here is, of course, on Training. In the five-year period 1963–68, federal expenditures for training increased 167 percent from $.3 to $.8 billion. However, the proportion of health expenditures allocated to training relative to total health expenditures in both years remained about the same—roughly 6.5 percent.

Approximately two-thirds of the 1968 training funds are earmarked for the Public Health Service, but an examination of the numbers of allied health personnel to be aided is very disappointing

[2] "Building America's Health," A Report to the President by the President's Commission on the Health Needs of the Nation in Vol. II: *America's Health Status, Needs, and Resources* (Washington, 1952), pp. 173–81.

[3] "Physicians for a Growing America," *Report of the Surgeon General's Consultant Group on Medical Education*, and "Toward Quality in Nursing Needs and Goals," *Report of the Surgeon General's Consultant Group on Nursing* (Washington, Dept. of Health, Education, and Welfare, 1959 and 1963).

[4] *Federal Health Programs, Special Analysis H* (Washington, Bureau of the Budget, January 1967).

both in absolute terms (1,200) and in relation to total Public Health Service manpower support (only 2.3 percent). Other federal departments having important medical manpower training programs are the Department of Defense ($75 million), the Department of Labor ($55 million), and the Veterans Administration ($39 million). The only other specific reference in the Budget to health manpower is the item concerning practical nurse training, under the aegis of the Department of Health, Education, and Welfare. Expenditures for this purpose were $7.5 million in 1966 and are scheduled to rise to $18.5 million in 1968, an increase of 146 percent in only two years.[5] This appears to represent a conscious attempt to cope with a general shortage of nursing services through the training of intermediate level nursing personnel.

Enabling Legislation and Its Implementation

As background material for the participants at a 1966 joint Department of Labor–Health, Education, and Welfare conference,[6] the Public Health Service identified and described briefly some sixty-four pieces of federal legislation, "affecting the supply and demand of health manpower" from 1956–1965, to which should be added the Allied Health Professions Personnel Training Act of 1966, and the Economic Opportunity Act of 1967, making for a total of sixty-six such laws enacted between 1956 and 1967.

We do not propose to duplicate that effort here. Rather we wish to comment on two of the programs—that under the Office of Education and that under the Department of Labor—as examples of the effect that some of these acts are having on the recruitment and training of allied health personnel.

[5] *Ibid.*, pp. 116 and 122. For a summary of VA programs, see W. M. Engle, "Solving the VA Health Shortage," *Employment Service Review* (November 1966), pp. 36–39.

[6] Dept. of Labor–Health, Education, and Welfare Conference, "Job Development and Training for Workers in Health Services: Background Data Book" (Washington, 1966), pp. 53–56.

Office of Education

In an annual report of the Office of Education the statement was made that, "During fiscal year 1964, the American system of vocational education was gearing up to meet the nation's changing manpower needs." [7] An analysis of the data presented in the body of that report, however, indicated that the achievements fell far short of the promise.

There are five major areas in which vocational and technical classes were provided in 1964: Agriculture, Distribution, Health, Home Economics, Technical and Trade, and Industry. Of a total enrollment of over 4.5 million, some 59,000 (or 1.3 percent) were in health occupations. Clearly, in light of all that has been presented above concerning the rapid growth of and the demand for health personnel, this distribution of enrollees is not compatible with the nation's manpower needs. Nor is this disappointing statistic due to lack of interest on the part of students. At one point the report states, for example, that "A medical assistant program in Wisconsin attracts three times as many applicants as can be accepted." Even within the small total, additional faults are evident: the enrollees are 97 percent female; and there is an especially low proportion of males at the secondary level—29 of 2,919 in practical nurse training, 9 of 300 in the dental assistant program, 2 of 289 in the medical assistant program, and 57 of 1,873 in "other health occupations." One of the most remarkable pieces of data in the report, and one that goes a long way to explain the deficiencies we have pointed out, is the fact that in 1964 only one state, Wisconsin, of the fifty-four states and areas, is listed as having expended any funds at all for vocational guidance in the health occupations—and it spent only $1,201.95. A major redirection in these programs is clearly indicated and even mandated by one of the enabling acts—

[7] *Vocational and Technical Education, Fiscal Year 1964* (Washington, Dept. of Health, Education, and Welfare, 1966), p. 3.

ograms rose to about 85,000 from the 59,000 noted above for)64. However, total enrollment in all of the programs also grew ith the result that the percentage in health occupations remained)out the same— a disappointing 1.4 percent. Data on expenditures :r health trainee in these programs present a more hopeful pic- re. In 1957 combined federal, state, and local expenditures per ainee enrolled in health curriculums was $47; by 1966 this figure id risen to $258. If the rise in expenditures per trainee is a mea- re of increased quality of the training, this would offset to some iall degree the low quantitative indexes that we have highlighted.[10]

epartment of Labor

When compared to the Office of Education programs, those ider the aegis of the Manpower Development and Training Act of)62 fare somewhat better, as far as the training of health man-)wer is concerned.

Between August, 1962, and September, 1965, 48,071 trainees id been approved for the health occupations—9.3 percent of all)provals over that period. Somewhat more than a year later, i.e.,)m August, 1962, to December, 1966, the cumulative total in the alth occupations rose to 63,036, a 50 percent increase.[11] In rela- 'e terms, health occupations rose to 10.5 percent of the new tal.

Some interesting facts emerge when one looks at the data for a mple year, instead of on a cumulative basis. In 1965, for exam- e, a total of 13,271 individuals received training in three identi- ible health occupations—licensed practical nurse, nurse's aide, id orderly.[12] This total represented 6.1 percent of all the trainees

[10] Calculated from data in letter from Grant Vernon, Associate Commissioner, pt. of Health, Education, and Welfare, to author, November 22, 1967.
[11] "Training under the MDTA for Health Occupations" (Washington, Dept. of bor, Office of Manpower Policy, Evaluation, and Research, n.d.). *Manpower port of the President, 1967*, p. 191.
[12] *Manpower Report of the President, 1966*, Table F-1, p. 219.

the Vocational Education Act of 1963—under
education programs are to be geared to labor ma

One of the strongest of the Office of Education
grams is that in practical nursing. The Health
of 1956 amended the basic Vocational Education
(George-Barden Act) by adding to the latter, Title
vides for federal grants to states of $5 million
matching basis) for "vocational Education in
Training." The term "practical nursing" was broad
clude "training of a similar nature which is design
uals engaged or preparing to engage in other healt
hospitals and other health agencies for such occu
examination of the distribution of enrollees under
1964 indicated that 71 percent were in the practica
percent were in the dental assistant groups, 6.1 per
cal assistant classes, and 15.4 percent in "other
tions" (included in this last group are dental lal
cians, dispensing opticians, medical laboratory as
unit management assistants, nurse's aides, operating
physical therapy assistants, and X-ray assistants).[9]

The 1956 amendments are noteworthy here as
explicit involvement of the federal government (a
matching feature to states and municipalities) in th
lied health manpower. This is a program which, fr
view of health manpower needs, has real potential ar
therefore be encouraged by removal of the inadeq
federal funds ceiling. Further, through the mounting
tive guidance program, particularly at the seconda
greater proportions of students (and more males esp
be directed toward the "other health occupations"
gram.

By 1966, total health enrollees in these vocation

[8] *Ibid.*, pp. 14, Table 19, p. 60, and p. 4.   [9] *Ibid.*, Table

in institutional and on-the-job training programs in that year. Even were we to add to these an additional 20 percent (derived from the cumulative data) in such health occupations as psychiatric aide, surgical technician, medical laboratory assistant, and dental assistant, occupations not separately identified in the data under review but which are undoubtedly included in the "professional and technical" category, the proportion of health to total trainees rises to 7.4 percent. Admittedly, this is higher than the 1.3 percent we found in the vocational education program, but it is also lower than the latter in absolute numbers—59,000 trainees in the Office of Education programs (in 1964) and 15,985 in the MDTA programs in 1965.

On a cumulative basis again, i.e., 1962–1966, some 50,000 trainees (LPN and nurse's aide) were enrolled in institutional (schools) courses and only 6,400 aides and orderlies were trained on-the-job training programs.[13] The on-job-training share of the trainees appears to be too low in view of the demonstrated effectiveness of these programs for the lower and even intermediate skill level occupations.

The occupational direction of the program likewise appears to be less than satisfactory. Over the period 1962 to 1966, fully 80 percent of all trainees were in the licensed practical nurse and nurse's aide categories and 11.2 percent and .7 percent respectively were in the specialized technical aide and health-clerical occupations (Table 7.2). The technical group is one that should for many obvious reasons, receive far greater support.

Better balances are also indicated in the demographic aspects of the program. For example, women constituted almost 90 percent of the trainees who were enrolled in the institutional course. A concerted effort should certainly be made to raise the male proportion especially in those jobs (mostly of a technical nature) where the traditional taboos against males are weakest.

[13] *Manpower Report of the President, 1967,* Table F-2, p. 277.

Table 7.2

Distribution of Authorized MDTA Trainees in
Health Occupations, August, 1962–December, 1966

Occupation	Number	*Percent* *Distribution*
Total	63,036	100.0
Professional nurse (refresher training)	4,723	7.5
Licensed practical nurse	20,695	32.8
Nurse's aide, orderly, and related occupations	30,028	47.6
Nurse's aide, orderly	27,220	
Clinical assistant	120	
Home attendant	448	
Housekeeper (medical service)	1,654	
Ward maid	378	
Other attendant	208	
Specialized technical aides	7,123	11.3
Dental technician	491	
Dentists' assistant	765	
Medical laboratory assistant	544	
Medical records aide	151	
Medical technician	147	
Occupational therapy aide	145	
Psychiatric aide	2,978	
Special diet worker	440	
Surgical technician	925	
X-ray technician	132	
Other	405	
Health clerical	467	.7
Ward clerk	320	
Secretary and other	147	

Source: *Manpower Report of the President, 1967*, Table 4, p. 191.

While the percentage of persons over 45 years of age being trained in health occupations is greater than that in all of the programs—14 percent to 10 percent respectively—a greater effort to enroll more older persons should nevertheless be made. And on the other end of the age scale, those below 19 years of age also appear to be underrepresented—only 10.7 percent of all health trainees.

The racial composition of the health trainees reveals imbalances that call for corrective action. Whereas 30 percent of all MDTA trainees are nonwhite, only 10 percent of the health trainees are nonwhite. Moreover, nonwhites constituted almost half of the persons receiving training as orderlies. A strong effort needs to be made then, not only to bring more nonwhites into the health occupations but also into the more skilled and better paying ones. An important impediment here, of course, is the question of educational levels. Trainees in the health occupations show higher levels of educational attainment than do all MDTA enrollees. In part, higher educational qualifications are required for the more advanced types of training, but it is also true, as MDTA pointed out, that there may be, "unnecessarily high educational requirements placed on subprofessional jobs by employers in the health field." [14] MDTA officials should strive by joint conferences with employers to develop more realistic standards for the jobs and, perhaps by demonstration projects, to show that high quality work (including lower turnover rates) is obtainable from trainees with less than the prescribed educational levels. This would be a real service to the entire health manpower field.

To date, the results of MDTA programs in health as measured by the post-training employment rates are of a mixed sort. On the one hand, the employment rates for licensed practical nurse trainees is excellent—it is 90 percent compared to the average of 74 percent for all institutional trainees. On the other hand, the rate for nurse's aides and ward attendants was 71 percent, or 3 percent less than the average. In view of the undiminished demand for these occupations, this is difficult to understand, but without the necessary data it is not possible to assess the reasons for this record.

MDTA includes the occupational training aspects of the now expired Area Redevelopment Act. As of June 30, 1965, about 15 percent (6,503 people) of enrollees under this program were in the

[14] "Training Under MDTA," p. 4.

health occupations. The problems here are two-fold: training is given to unemployed or underemployed in depressed areas; and there is a statutory limitation of sixteen weeks as the maximum duration for training courses. On the first point, depressed areas in general are not overly endowed with large health facilities, so that unless provision is made for the establishment of new facilities such as neighborhood health centers and clinics, opportunities for employment in the area will be limited. Second, the sixteen-week ceiling is insufficient time for learning many health jobs and virtually relegates the ARA segment to a nurse's aide program exclusively. Given the difficulties experienced by MDTA in the nurse's aide field just cited, the program in this form warrants serious re-consideration.

This brief review of two major federal (or federal plus state and local) programs leads us to believe that too much of the training is, as one writer put it, "training for the short run, the local area or dead-end occupations." [15] But the positive aspects of the program should also be pointed out. Even though these programs are insufficient in amount and often misdirected, thousands of health workers are getting training through them—training which either is not or has not been available elsewhere, or if available, is not of good quality, or is costly both in direct fees and in foregone earnings. Moreover, a good part of the blame for the relatively poor representation in the health occupations must be placed on the historical performance of the health field itself for manpower below the autonomous levels. As we have detailed throughout this book, and as the most recent Manpower Report of the President pointed out: "The foremost reason for the current personnel shortages is economic—jobs in the health industry generally offer lower pay and less attractive employment conditions than other fields of work calling for

[15] Harold L. Wilensky, "Careers, Counseling, and the Curriculum," *Journal of Human Resources,* Vol. II, No. 1 (Winter 1967), p. 36.

comparable educational preparation. Low wages and salaries, coupled with a general lack of career advancement opportunities and many problems with respect to working conditions, make it difficult for hospitals and nursing homes to attract or retain efficient workers." [16]

There are signs, however, that new ways of reaching out to the population, new job categories, and experimentation with new institutional forms are serving to remedy some of the defects noted. For example, the Neighborhood Youth Corps has been training disadvantaged youth for jobs as ward attendants, orderlies, X-ray technician aides, and dental technician aides as well as for various clerical and maintenance positions. Also noteworthy, and dovetailing with the program just mentioned, is the fact that "A significant national contract with a nonprofit agency, the Association of Rehabilitation Centers, will provide for training—upgrading and entry—for 900 persons in nonprofessional occupations to help alleviate the shortages in rehabilitation hospitals and related institutions. The trainees will be recruited from among the disadvantaged and wherever possible, from those who have had preliminary work experience in the health field under NYC (Neighborhood Youth Corps) programs." [17]

Another extremely interesting and imaginative item, important more for its implications for the future than for the numbers currently involved, concerns a union initiated joint undertaking by the Merchant Marine, the U.S. Public Health Service, and the Department of Labor under MDTA, for the training of a new occupational category—purser–pharmacist mate. Termed "the first large group of medical middlemen," these graduates from a nine-month training program will provide some modicum of medical care to ship personnel on nonmilitary vessels, who formerly had none

[16] *Manpower Report of the President, 1967*, p. 190.
[17] *Ibid.*, pp. 191 and 58.

available to them. J. M. Michael, an assistant Surgeon General, called the school "a model and a pattern for providing medical skills short of full-fledged professional standards to such agencies as the Peace Corps, the Agency for International Development and the Bureau of Indian Affairs." [18]

We cannot leave the subject of training without commenting on the recently enacted Allied Health Professions Personnel Training Act of 1966, which was briefly noted earlier. Previous federal legislation dealing directly with health manpower such as the Health Professions Educational Assistance Act of 1963, the Nurse Training Act of 1964, the Graduate Public Health Training Amendments of 1964, and the Health Professions Educational Assistance Amendments of 1965, was concerned primarily with the "professional" level occupations: physician, dentist, nurse, podiatrist, and optometrist. The 1966 act, for the first time, focused on other so-called "allied" health professions, that is to say, the many medical workers who are required to have a baccalaureate degree as a minimum (see Chapters 1 and 2). Congress was (correctly, we think) persuaded to include the junior colleges as well under the legislation so that with the exception of the practical nurse and aide–orderly–clerk positions, we have here basically an act dealing with allied health manpower.

The impetus for the new act stemmed from the conviction that

as health care becomes more complex, and as demands for health care increase, all of the functions of care cannot be performed by the doctors and dentists themselves. The supply of doctors, dentists and other highly trained professionals simply cannot be expanded sufficiently to meet these needs. A large number of allied professional and technical workers will be required to extend the reach of physicians and dentists. Looking ahead 10 years we can see that the supply of physicians will even then be about the same as it is today in relation to the population. Our hopes and needs to provide the best in health care for the American

[18] The New York *Times,* June 29, 1967, p. 85.

people can be fulfilled only to the extent that it is possible to increase the numbers and capabilities of allied health workers.[19]

Proponents of this legislation projected an increase in the capacity of existing schools of 3 to 4,000 allied health workers annually. This would be accomplished in a three-year program concentrating on the following four areas: grants for construction of teaching facilities; grants to schools for educational improvements; traineeships to help prepare teachers, administrators, supervisors, and other personnel in specialized practice; and project grants to develop, demonstrate, or evaluate curriculums for training new types of health technologists. New funds for health manpower training functions (apart from the student loan provisions) were projected to be $8 million in 1967, $18 million in 1968, and $26 million in 1969.[20]

As can be seen from the foregoing, the thrust of the act is on teacher training of allied health manpower and it thus represents a longer-run investment whose yield will increase over time. The addition of the junior college or associate degree programs also provides for a more immediate increase in the supply of technical health personnel. Another far-reaching facet of the legislation is that implicit as well as explicit support is given to interdisciplinary training of health manpower.

It is too early to assess the results of this program. From our viewpoint, it represents a new and correct turn in the attempts by the federal government to increase—directly and indirectly—the supply of allied health manpower and thereby to increase the effectiveness of health manpower as a whole.

The act could be strengthened by extending the "student loan forgiveness" and "guaranteed loan" provisions to all of the occupa-

[19] Report of the Committee on Interstate and Foreign Commerce on H.R. 13196, *Allied Health Professions Personnel Training Act of 1966*, House Report No. 1682, 89C2, June 16, 1966, p. 6.
[20] Hears./89C2 CIFC/March 29–31, 1966, pp. 19, 42, and 23.

tions covered in it, something which it does not now do explicitly. Second, in order to encourage even further a more equitable regional distribution of manpower, relocation loans or subsidies might well be included.

As important as the new emphasis on allied health manpower is, of even greater importance is the recognition by the proponents of this legislation of the dynamic processes at work in the provision of health services. In the words of the House committee which studied the bill:

The development of technology in the medical and dental fields carries with it the necessity of developing new types of personnel. Expanding scientific knowledge and methodology are creating a situation which demands a flexible approach to the training of auxiliary personnel in the health occupations. New kinds of specially trained technologists and technicians will be required in the laboratories as new procedures and techniques of diagnosis and treatment are developed. *There are unknown quantities in the organization of health services for the future; today's job descriptions may not be tomorrow's.*

The committee considered it particularly important that grants be available to educational institutions for the continuing development of methods of training health personnel at this level, to match the continually changing technology and organization of health care.[21] [Emphasis ours]

Many other federal activities affect allied health manpower as a part of their on-going programs. In fiscal 1965, for example, over $10 million was provided by the National Institute of Mental Health to support training for graduate social work students, and $6.4 million for psychologists, many of them in the medical field.[22] Programs primarily directed elsewhere—medical research, com-

[21] Report on H.R. 13196, p. 19.
[22] "Training Grant Program, Fiscal Year 1965: A Statistical Sourcebook," *Public Health Service Publication No. 1521* (Washington, National Institute of Mental Health).

munity services, demonstration projects—include training of personnel at all levels as part of their mandate.

More specifically, the 1967 amendments to the Social Security Act (the "Harris" amendments) require the states to provide for the training and effective use of paid subprofessional staff as community service aides, many of whom will be in the health services.

An important new act which may have a great potential impact on subprofessional health training is the Economic Opportunity Act of 1967, particularly Part B of Title I (the Scheuer amendment), which is considered the authorizing legislation for the so-called, "New Careers" program. Section 123 of this act enables the director to provide financial assistance for "special programs which provide unemployed or low income persons with jobs leading to career opportunities . . . in health, education, welfare, neighborhood redevelopment and public safety . . . (and) which give promise of contributing to the broader adoption of new methods of structuring jobs and new methods of providing job ladder opportunities and which provide opportunities for further occupational training to facilitate career advancement."

Although education and training are important aspects of the supply of allied health personnel, and absorb most of the federal funds allocated, other areas of importance to manpower—recruitment, employment, utilization, and data collection—receive attention from a variety of government sources.

Efforts in recruitment are mainly limited to the dissemination of information to guidance counselors, employment service counselors, or to interested individuals about the opportunities and requirements for health occupations. The *Occupational Outlook Handbook* of BLS, and the *Health Careers Guidebook* of the U.S. Employment Service are widely used sources of career information. Direct recruitment through exhortation and advertisement is largely left to the professional societies and the employers although every government-sponsored training program must perforce "recruit" its own trainees, and every state employment service counselor who finds a job in a hospital for an unspecialized worker in effect "recruits" a health service worker.

The aspect of career information dissemination, whether governmental or nongovernmental, which deserves attention is the tendency to upgrade the published job requirements to the point that, from a reading of the literature, one would conclude that every health worker in a hospital was registered with a professional society and that even the least-skilled manual worker possessed a high-school diploma. The reason for this paper upgrading is clear—the agencies involved have an obligation to try to raise the quality of health workers and the education of the citizens. Yet it may be questioned whether this upgrading helps to relieve the shortage of workers or to enable prospective workers to find jobs.

Closely related to recruitment efforts are employment efforts. The main agency here is, of course, the U.S. Employment Service and the affiliated state employment services, which provide job-finding assistance to prospective workers. Although the state employment services provide the majority of the formal employment contacts, their place in the total scheme is somewhat limited by the nature of the allied health labor market, in which job information is mainly disseminated through word of mouth, newspaper advertisements, and personal contact. Federal funds are increasingly being allocated to assist in matching workers with jobs (e.g., the job vacancy statistics program) and in persuading trained housewives (nurses and technologists) to return to work.

Some experimental and demonstration projects on utilization have taken place through the various agencies of the Department of Labor and the Public Health Service, but direct effects are limited. Allied health manpower utilization, by its nature, is more likely to be studied as part of the larger number of projects concerning hospital organization or medical, dental or nursing manpower.

The collection of statistical data is an important part of the government's activities. The Bureau of the Census, the Bureau of Labor Statistics, and the Bureau of Employment Security have ongoing responsibility for the collection of occupational and industrial data. In addition, such efforts as the *Health Manpower Source Books* and the recent American Hospital Association survey of hospital employment, both under the Public Health Service, are an important addition to information in the area. In many cases, data gathered by the government are the only data available for analysis. In all too many cases, no data are available at all.

Summary

As with other governmental programs, health manpower programs and projects often suffer from interagency competition, excessive administrative layers, duplication, delays in refunding, and other such bureaucratic ills.[23] One writer, for example, reporting on community training experiences in a certain city, remarked: "Unfortunately, in this city there are three separate agencies under three separate Federal Government grants which are training the same level health worker. The agencies do cooperate, but they do not coordinate their programs."[24]

Levitan and Mangum point out that the hub of the coordination problem lies in multiple federal funding sources. These in turn, can be made more manageable by the use of joint funding (one or more federal funding sources transfer funds to a single agency which acts as sponsor of a local project) and coupled contracts (negotiations

[23] Sar A. Levitan and Garth L. Mangum, "Making Sense of Federal Manpower Policy," *Policy Papers in Human Resources and Industrial Relations No. 2* (University of Michigan and Wayne State University, Institute of Labor and Industrial Relations, March 1967), pp. 13–14.

[24] "Training Health Service Workers: The Critical Challenge," *Proceedings of the Dept. of Labor–Dept. of Health, Education, and Welfare Conference of Job Development and Training for Workers in Health Services* (Washington, February 14–17, 1966), p. 56.

by a local agency with a number of funding sources for the operation of a single project). The authors cite an interesting application of the coupled funds technique in the health manpower area: "In a Detroit hospital . . . ward clerk trainees are selected from welfare rolls, provided basic education and institutional skill training in school facilities and then enter on-the-job training at the hospital. . . . Involved are separate contracts drawing funds from adult basic education, work experience and MDTA, both institutional and OJT." [25]

The creation of the new Bureau of Health Manpower in the Public Health Service should go far to strengthen federal programs in this area. By acting as a focal point for the coordination of interdepartmental and interagency programs, this bureau has the potential of eliminating duplication, as well as of providing initiative for new program directions. Hopefully the bureau will be given broad operational scope, adequate funds, and required staff to carry out its functions.

The largest portion of governmental assistance to allied health manpower is in the form of funds to assist education and training. Since people are the main means of production of health services, and since allied health workers are in relatively short supply, this appears to be a rational allocation of governmental resources. However, the importance of governmental support in other areas should not be overlooked.

We agree, for instance, with a statement in the recently published report of the National Advisory Manpower Commission on Health Manpower, to wit: "The scarcity of capital funds for improving hospital operations is a major factor in the present wasteful use of health manpower. Because labor costs are 60–70 percent of hospital operating expenses, there is great potential for conserving resources by upgrading facilities through capital investment." [26]

[25] Levitan and Mangum, p. 19.

[26] *Report of the National Advisory Commission on Health Manpower*, I (November 1967), 60.

Federal support for hospital construction via the Hill-Burton Act has indeed been an important factor in the expansion of health facilities since 1948. This legislation perhaps may be extended to the modernization of obsolete facilities and to the support of architectural experimentation and innovation with the goal of a more efficient combination of labor and capital for the production and distribution of health services.

CHAPTER 8

Overview and Recommendations

IN THE following summary we wish to do three things: present the major propositions and findings arising from our research; present some guidelines derived from our study for allied health manpower policies; and indicate areas where additional research is needed.

Major Propositions and Findings

Health manpower is growing in absolute terms as well as in relation to the total labor force. Simultaneously, the health manpower "mix"—that is, the relative proportion of allied health to total health manpower—is undergoing rapid change in the non-core direction for a variety of reasons, chief among which are supply deficiencies, advances in the state of the medical art, technical innovations, and cost pressures. The data we have examined indicate that these factors are of greater force than opposing trends such as automation or other technological changes. More than 80 percent of total health manpower falls into the category of allied health manpower as we have defined it.

The hospital, as the major type of employing institution, currently exerts the strongest influence over wages, hours, and working conditions of allied health personnel.

In a regional sample of fifteen SMSAs, we found that the growth in hospital employment exceeded aggregate employment growth rates in each area, although there were wide inter-area differentials in the hospital personnel to population ratios.

Instead of there being a single homogeneous labor market for allied health personnel, there exists a collection of smaller, quasi-independent submarkets composed of the separate and rigidly defined occupations. At the lower-skill levels, these markets tend to be local and regional in scope; at the higher levels there exist national labor markets.

Evidence of general and specific shortages of health manpower was found in the following types of labor market adjustments over the 1956–66 decade: rapid wage increases, more nonwhites, intra- and inter-regional changes in relative wage structures.

Health service workers are predominantly female, and the female proportion shows little sign of decreasing in recent years. Efforts to increase the recruitment of males are likely to falter unless the work is made more attractive in terms of wages and career opportunities. The growth of nonnursing, especially the technical occupations, has opened more supervisory positions to males, but the small size of the employing unit and the fact that there is no administrative hierarchy separate from the professional hierarchy prevent extensive upward mobility and inhibit male employment.

The charitable and nonprofit background of hospitals has adversely affected attitudes toward capital and manpower and toward the utilization of the human resources of the industry. This factor helps explain, but does not justify, the relatively low wages and poor working conditions that were and are prevalent. Recent changes in legislation such as Fair Labor Standards Act coverage, a new tone of militancy by many professional organizations, the growth of unions, as well as general shortages of manpower, are all combining to bring hospital wages more in line with those of other industries. Simultaneously, public pressure to keep costs low while increasing services has made the industry more aware of the importance of efficient utilization of manpower.

One of the most important barriers to optimum utilization of allied health personnel is the extreme specialization of workers and the overly rigid separation between types of workers. This is reinforced by professional organizations of each type of worker, by separate training facilities, and by outdated laws and anachronistic customs. Among the consequences of this malutilization are dead-end occupations, high turnover rates, job dissatisfaction, and higher operating costs.

The excessive turnover rates in the health services are partly due to the utilization of large numbers of women, married or unmarried, who are more likely than men to change jobs for noncareer-related reasons. More importantly, the location of the major work units, the hospitals, are scattered throughout the country; there are a large number of occupations required per unit and relatively few workers of a given occupation per unit. The lack of promotion or transfer opportunities within the small units necessitates the worker's quitting his job and moving to another location to improve his income, job assignment, or working conditions.

The diffused location and relatively small size of the employing units requires that the training facilities be likewise diffused and quite small for each occupation. Hence the economies of scale possible in larger training institutions are not realized. The training units are most likely to be merged with other units—hospitals, vocational schools, or colleges. Increased demands for health services, together with changes in job content and classification, have made it both feasible and advisable to train larger numbers of students in "allied health professions" schools or, as they are sometimes called, schools of "related health occupations."

The training of allied health personnel, which until recent years took place largely within hospitals, is increasingly moving away from the hospital and toward educational institutions at all levels, both public and private. The education and training of allied health workers is gradually but surely coming to be viewed as a public education responsibility by the large metropolitan areas. As newer occupations emerge from the work setting, however, their training should remain within the hospital until the requirements of the job become sufficiently standardized and the numbers to be trained become sufficiently large to justify the formalization of the training programs and their transfer to educational institutions.

Formal training within educational institutions tends to be longer than hospital-based training, with greater emphasis on general education and on theory. This has the disadvantage of extending the time and expense of training and of requiring that the trainee be academically oriented. On the other hand, the integration of allied health training into the general educational system enables the worker to receive academic credit for his training. Academic credit can be transferred to other institutions, and can serve as a basis for further education and training in the same or in different fields.

At present, the majority of health workers have less than four years of education or training after high school. The prerequisite educational level for the vast majority of allied health training or education is expected to be no less than and no more than high-school graduation. This in itself limits the potential supply of workers. Furthermore, a high proportion of health workers do not enter training directly after graduation but two, five, ten, and even twenty years later. Despite this, most recruitment efforts and training programs are directed to the graduating senior.

Professionalization is only partially successful due to the lack of independent status of the various occupations. Professionalization helps to raise the skill levels of the workers and to provide standardization of training and skills throughout the country. Professional societies strive to instill in their members "pride of craftsmanship." On the other hand, professionalization also attempts to decrease the flow of workers from alternative sources, and erects barriers to occupational mobility. Each profession attempts to improve its own position at the expense of others, and interprofessional jealousy is not unusual.

Guidelines for Policies

Although, as we have seen, allied health wage rates have risen rapidly from 1956 to 1966, wage levels are still too low to attract many females (who can earn more as stenographers) and they are still less of an inducement to males who may have to support families. The $1.00 minimum wage for hospital and nursing home workers effective in 1967, and which is to rise slowly to $1.60 in 1971, is insufficient and should be amended upward if it is to function as an effective recruiting and retaining mechanism.

The movement to include all health service workers under the unemployment insurance and workmen's compensation laws should be hastened.

In the area of labor–management relations, it is imperative that procedures for orderly collective bargaining be developed in order to avoid work stoppages, which, in the health field, are paticularly onerous and embarrassing to all parties.

More effective job information channels are needed. The Nurses and Medical Placement offices of the state employment services appear to be the logical focal points for gathering and disseminating such information as well as for providing aptitude and achievement tests and for screening applicants and checking references. State and local Health Career councils can be of great help in this effort.

Greater efforts need to be made to attract more males, more nonwhite, and more part-time workers.

Recruitment efforts should be expanded and aimed at high-school graduates who do not wish to continue along the academic route, to older women who wish to work but who lack previous educational requirements, and to junior high-school students who are headed for the general rather than the academic secondary school track.

The new educational institutions known as "Schools of the Allied Health Professions" should receive widespread support. Every effort should be made to have one such school attached to each medical school so that medical students may be educated in their formative years to understand the functions of and to learn to work with non-core personnel. These schools would also demonstrate the value of a "core curriculum" which would be common to all allied health students and would make for greater occupational inter-changeability.

Support should be given to the development of new forms of health facilities utilizing the "indigenous nonprofessionals" in urban neighborhoods as well as in rural areas.

The National Committee on Employment of Youth, however, has issued some well-advised words of caution in this regard. In a recent study they pointed out that: "When subprofessionals are seen as an expedient, made necessary by shortages of professionals, then the jobs usually are inherently temporary and the least important and demanding ones in the judgment of the professionals. When the subprofessional concept is equated with providing jobs for the poor, the jobs are similarly limited in scope, are temporary or make work, because the emphasis is on income for the worker, with job integrity a secondary consideration. And from both points of view, job creation is most often restricted to attempts to fit subprofessional jobs into or around the existing structures." [1]

Federal legislation, such as the Allied Health Professions Personnel Training Act of 1966, should cover the whole spectrum of allied health manpower, be extended beyond the three year mandate, and have more adequate funding. Similarly, the recommendation on the Training of Health Technicians by the President's Commission on Heart Disease, Cancer, and Stroke is particularly noteworthy and deserving of support.

[1] Edith F. Lynton, "The Subprofessional: From Concepts to Careers." Report of a Conference to Expand and Develop Subprofessional Roles in Health, Education, and Welfare conducted by the National Committee on Employment of Youth (New York, Sept. 30, 1967), p. 11.

Specifically, "The Commission [recommended] greatly increased effort and investment in the recruitment and training of health technicians and other paramedical personnel whose skills are essential to the control of heart disease, cancer, and stroke"; and further, "The supply of health manpower to support a full-scale attack on heart disease, cancer, and stroke can be recruited and developed only if full use is made of existing programs and authorities, especially those which can recruit into the ancillary health disciplines persons not normally attracted into health pursuits, including the economically disadvantaged and technologically displaced, the handicapped and the elder citizens." [2]

MDTA, Vocational Education, and Office of Economic Opportunity programs require expansion and, as was pointed out in Chapter 7, redirection toward occupations as well as toward population groups not now covered or inadequately represented. An equitable allocation of funds for allied health personnel should also be provided for the Scheuer–Nelson Subprofessional Career Act.

Closer coordination and liaison should be developed among agencies such as the Bureau of Health Manpower of the Public Health Service, the Intra-departmental Committee on Health Manpower of the Department of Labor, and the President's Committee on Health Manpower.

Important problems surrounding the employment and utilization of allied health personnel have their roots in hospital management. Physicians, unaware of labor market factors, often set unreasonable and unrealistic standards for non-core personnel, thus complicating the task of the personnel department. The alternative here must be to reorganize a given department (service) along more rational lines so that many functions can be performed by personnel without college degrees. In addition, a greater centralization of the hiring function in professional personnel departments is needed. A strong

[2] "A National Program to Conquer Heart Disease, Cancer and Stroke" (Washington, 1964), I, 60–61.

and well-oriented hospital management can do a great deal to achieve a more optimum utilization of both core and non-core health personnel and can do much in promoting policies to reduce turnover rates.

In the same vein, since laboratory tests, X-rays, diagnostic instrumentation, and therapeutic and rehabilitation facilities have all expanded greatly in recent years, older hospitals, which were not designed for these functions, now provide wholly inadequate work environments for many allied health personnel. A large renovation program is obviously called for if optimum utilization and increased productivity of health personnel in obsolescent hospitals are to be realized. Similarly, new hospitals and health facilities must be designed with the increased role of "ancillary" functions given full recognition.

Just as continuing education is important for physicians, so is it equally important for other health personnel. Provision must be made either in the hospital or in educational institutions for periodic in-service educational upgrading.

The civilian sector should make much more use of veterans with health training. A great and probably measurable increase in the quality of medical care in this country would occur from the simple expedient of having a medical corpsman on every ambulance call. Not only would more appropriate action (or inaction, as the case may be) be taken on initially viewing the patient, but emergency measures could be applied while the patient is en route to the hospital.

It is particularly gratifying to note that in mid-October, 1967, the Department of Health, Education, and Welfare, the Department of Defense, the Veterans' Administration, and the Department of Labor initiated a major program known as Project Remed, designed to encourage former servicemen, trained in the health area, to enter civilian occupations through recruitment, retraining, and reemployment efforts.

Research Needs

Of utmost importance for continuing studies in this area are reliable current data on health manpower on a local basis. Even in a city like New York, there is no single agency that collects comprehensive data on health manpower.

Fundamental to economic analyses are data on incomes, broken down by occupational groups. These are not now available on a comprehensive, continuous basis.

The job vacancy statistics program of the Department of Labor, when expanded not only geographically but also occupationally, to include most if not all of the detailed health occupations, will provide crucial and much needed data. A corollary here, of course, is the necessity of more accurate and standardized job descriptions.

More demonstration projects utilizing different core and non-core staffing patterns are needed to yield information on optimum utilization and on productivity.

We need to identify more specifically than we have the legal and extra-legal barriers to geographic as well as to occupational mobility.

Studies on where hospital workers go when they voluntarily leave their jobs would be of great importance for the analysis of turnover rates as well as for mobility analysis in general.

Studies of job dissatisfaction among those currently employed would also reveal a great deal about internal hospital management problems as well as about allied health personnel in general—their organizations, their aspirations, and the like.

There are no reliable data on total student enrollment in the myriad educational institutions, both public and private, providing education and training of one sort or another.

An important attempt to fill this gap is provided by the "Survey of Schools and Programs in Health Occupations Education, 1964–

65." This survey, the first of its kind, was sponsored by the National Center for Educational Statistics and the Health Occupations Unit of the Division of Vocational and Technical Education in the Office of Education. This effort needs to be supplemented by other surveys which will include activities presently excluded such as: on-the-job training programs, nurse's-aide programs, baccalaureate and higher degree programs, and programs offered for profit.

Information on the amounts and proportions of nonregistered vs. registered health personnel currently employed is not now available on any comprehensive scale.

Although there is information readily available concerning the amount of education and training desired or required for the various occupations, there is almost no information on how much education the workers actually have, how much they actually need, or how much they actually utilize. Support for research in this area should be expanded.

More information from those programs that have been instituted as well as more pilot programs for the training of new types of allied health personnel such as physician assistants, the non-M.D., non-Ph.D. mental health therapists, male surgical technicians, pediatric and obstetric aides, and the like would be most useful.

The foregoing findings, propositions, and guidelines have not been presented in order of priority. They are the major trends and implications which emerged from our analysis and from our field interviews. Our primary goal throughout the study was to provide a firmer factual and conceptual base that could be used both for a better understanding of current allied health manpower problems and as guidelines for developing policies more appropriate to their long-run solution.

Index